OSTEOPOROSIS:
THE NUMBERS ARE ALARMING!

- 80 percent of women do not get enough calcium every day!
- After age 30, women tend to lose 1 percent of their bone mass every year—after menopause, this loss can jump to 4 percent a year!
- Men are 50 percent more likely to suffer a fracture due to osteoporosis than to develop prostate cancer!

IMPROVE *YOUR* ODDS!

Super Calcium Counter gives you everything you need to start building strong bones today:

- A personal risk–assessment test
- The 21-day bone-boosting food diary
- The latest on bone-building supplements and drugs
- The calcium counter that rates more than 2,000 foods and beverages
- Delicious recipes—from Walnut Muffins and Ginger Salmon to Orange Julius Smoothies—that provide calcium and all the other important bone-boosting nutrients

DON'T WAIT! USE THE POWER OF NUTRITION TO PREVENT OR REVERSE OSTEOPOROSIS!

SUPER CALCIUM COUNTER

The Essential Guide to Preventing Osteoporosis and Building Strong Bones

Harris McIlwain, M.D.,
and Debra Fulghum Bruce

Kensington Books
Kensington Publishing Corp.
http://www.kensingtonbooks.com

CONTENTS

ACKNOWLEDGMENTS

While there are many who gave time for this project, including our families, we are especially appreciative of Linda McIlwain for the many hours of research she contributed to this book project. Her enthusiasm and untiring dedication were steadfast, and for this, we are indebted.

Two other women deserve acknowledgment, as well. To Denise Marcil, our literary agent, we celebrate this book with you and thank you for your commitment to osteoporosis prevention. We also are grateful for the encouragement and unfailing dedication shown by our editor, Tracy Bernstein, as she made herself available to us during the writing stages. Others who helped to make this book possible include: Brittnye Bruce, Ashley Bruce, Michael McIlwain, Jan Mashburn, M.A., Hugh Cruse, M.S.P.H., Laura McIlwain, M.D., Kimberly McIlwain, M.D., and Alyn Gauthier. For all of these people and their talents, we are thankful.

ABBREVIATIONS AND SYMBOLS

BBR	bone-boosting requirements	*	not available
		mcg	microgram(s)
diam.	diameter	mg	milligram(s)
fl.	fluid	oz.	ounce(s)
g	gram(s)	lb.	pound(s)
"	inches	tbsp.	tablespoon(s)
IU	international units	tsp.	teaspoon(s)
<	less than	tr.	trace

vit A = vitamin A   mag = magnesium
vit C = vitamin C   phos = phosphorus
  cal = calcium   zinc = zinc

Section One

THE ESSENTIAL GUIDE TO BUILDING STRONG BONES

Keeping bones strong for an entire lifetime is possible *if* you become aware of the vitamins and minerals needed to prevent osteoporosis. In listing the nutrient values of the most common foods, we used the latest information provided by the United States Department of Agriculture (**USDA**), as well as extensive data from food producers, packagers, and distributors.

When you compare this information with packaging labels or other nutrition resources, the values may differ. These variations occur for many reasons, including regional and seasonal differences in produce and how the food is gathered, processed, stored, and shipped. *Do not* let this stop you from incorporating these bone-boosting foods into your daily meal plan.

We have listed foods in the following categories:

Beverages	Milk, Cream, and Yogurt
Breads, Flour, and Grains	Miscellaneous
Candies	Nuts, Seeds, and Butters
Cereals	Pasta, Noodles, and Rice
Cheeses	Poultry
Desserts and Toppings	Prepared Foods
Eggs	Salad
Fast Foods	Salad Dressings
Fats	Seafood
Fruit	Snack Foods
Fruit Juices	Soups
Gravies, Sauces, and Dips	Soy
Meats	Vegetables

Osteoporosis is a diagnosis that more than *half* of all women over age forty-five will hear in the near future. By age seventy-five, more than *one-third* of all men have this disease. Once thought to be a consequence of aging, we now know that osteoporosis is *not* a normal progression and can be prevented.

Yet why is osteoporosis such a growing concern? Let's look at some bone-chilling facts:

- *Thirty million* Americans have osteoporosis at this time; *80 percent* are women and *less than 10 percent* are diagnosed.
- Women have a *one-in-two chance* of fracturing a bone due to osteoporosis in their lifetime—fractures that can lead to disability, disfigurement, and even death.
- A woman's risk of hip fracture is *equal* to her *combined risk* of breast, uterine, and ovarian cancer.
- *Menopause* is the single most important cause of osteoporosis due to the effect on bone of decreased levels of estrogen.
- Men are *50 percent* more likely to fracture a bone due to osteoporosis than to get prostate cancer. By age seventy-five, *one in four* men will suffer a broken hip and *one in seven* will have a spinal fracture.

The figures are startling. After osteoporosis quietly weakens your bones over the years, even normal stress on bones— such as sitting, standing, coughing, or hugging a loved one— can cause fractures that lead to chronic pain and immobility. After more fractures, osteoporosis may cause deformities, crippling, and even death.

Osteoporosis operates silently. It can start early in life and leaves no warning signs until a fracture occurs. A Washington, D.C. corporation recently gave bone density tests to all female employees and found that, among women ages forty to fifty, a startling *56 percent* had lower than normal bone density, and *19 percent* had bone density scores which indicated almost guaranteed future osteoporosis.

The good news is that osteoporosis can be prevented if you start today to *THINK BONE!* In fact, it is never too soon or too late to start keeping bones strong. With the extraordinary breakthroughs in diagnosis, prevention, and treatment of osteoporosis, almost everyone can now live fracture-free.

A simple bone density test, such as DXA (dual-energy X-ray absorptiometry), gives doctors a guaranteed way to detect this disease years *before* the first fracture occurs. This simple and inexpensive test is done in your doctor's office, and many insurance companies will cover the cost. If the test shows that your bone density is low, and you are at risk for fractures, your doctor can start you on a bone-strengthening program. This will include adding bone-boosting foods, weight-bearing and strength-training exercises, and taking bone-building medications and estrogen (for women) that actually reverse bone loss and increase bone density.

Fosamax (alendronate) is one of several new medications for use in the treatment of osteoporosis. Through numerous tests, these medications have been proven to significantly increase bone density. Over a one- to three-year period, people on this type of medication have had increases in bone density of 6 percent or more. In fact, studies show more than 90 percent of all patients respond to treatment with these medications.

Ages, Stages, and Risk Factors

Age and Bone Loss

The most critical time to build bone is during childhood and the teenage years. At this time, more bone is built than removed, so bones become larger and stronger. Recent studies reveal that 90 percent of total bone mass in females may already be in place by age sixteen. In fact, when a girl gets her first menstrual period during puberty, bone mass is increasing at its highest pace. But instead of taking advantage of building bones while the body is ''in the mood,'' the average teenage girl gets only about *300 to 800 mg* of bone-boosting calcium a day (the optimal requirement for teenage girls is *1,300–1,500 mg* a day—the equivalent of more than four glasses of milk).

If our bodies could continue to build bone throughout our

lifetimes, osteoporosis would not be a problem. Yet at some point, usually in their mid-thirties, women begin to lose bone at the rate of 1 percent per year (men's bone loss usually occurs five to ten years later in life). At this time, more bone is removed than built, and osteoporosis starts throughout the skeleton. Because of hormonal changes during menopause, bone loss jumps to *about 4 percent per year* during the five to ten years after menopause (usually ages forty-five to fifty-five). Women may lose bone faster during these years than any other period. For those who didn't drink milk or eat bone-boosting foods during childhood and adolescence, or for those with several risk factors, such as cigarette smoking or lack of regular exercise, the rate is even higher.

The Stages of Osteoporosis

Understanding the stages of osteoporosis will enable you to see how bone loss and physical changes occur over time. While Stages 1 and 2 are still without any visible symptoms, it is during these stages that prevention of bone loss using the bone-boosting measures in this guide is most effective.

Stage 1 usually begins after ages thirty to thirty-five. There are no symptoms, no signs, and no detection using bone density tests. Bone removal begins to outpace bone formation.

Stage 2 usually occurs after age thirty-five. While there are no symptoms and no signs, detection is now possible using bone density tests.

Stage 3 usually occurs after age forty-five. At this stage, bones have become thin enough to result in fractures. Detection can be made using bone density tests.

Stage 4 occurs at age fifty-five and older. Not only will you have more fractures, but pain and deformity may now result. Detection is made through X rays and bone density tests.

Are You at Risk?

There are specific genetic and environmental risk factors that set the stage for bone loss. While these factors do not cause the disease, they can alert you to an underlying problem. Some of the risk factors—such as your age, sex, race, and family history—cannot be controlled. For example, Caucasian women are at higher risk than African-American women. Likewise, if your mother and grandmother had osteoporosis, your chances are greatly increased. Nonetheless, there are many factors over which you do have control, and these are the ones you can focus on changing.

—**Sex**

Women get osteoporosis about ten to fifteen years earlier than men. You cannot control this risk factor, so be sure to change the ones you can.

—**Family history**

If someone in your family has osteoporosis, especially your mother, sister, or grandmother, this places you at a much greater risk. Make important lifestyle changes for prevention.

—**Race**

If you are a Caucasian or Asian female, this places you at a higher risk for bone loss and resulting fractures. Knowing this, eliminate other risk factors.

—**Menopause or other loss of menstrual periods (amenorrhea)**

The decline of estrogen during menopause makes bone more susceptible to osteoporosis. Talk with your doctor about your specific needs, and see if supplemental estrogen may help keep your bones strong. Estrogen is still the main effective protective measure for osteoporosis after menopause. If you have abnormal loss of menstrual periods from strenuous exercise, check with your doctor to see if your exercise routine should be modified or if medications should be added.

—**Underweight and/or petite frame**

People who are underweight and who have a petite frame are at a higher risk for osteoporosis. Be sure to maintain a healthy weight, eating nutritious bone-boosting foods and exercising to keep bones strong.

—A diet low in calcium and vitamin D

Studies reveal that more than 90 percent of all women and 60 percent of all men get too little calcium to keep bones strong. Recently, the government has identified low calcium intake as one of the major nutritional problems in the United States today. Many people, especially women, avoid dairy products to save calories and stay slim. Some do not use dairy products because of lactose intolerance. If this applies to you, be sure you get ample calcium and vitamin D in your diet from other bone-boosting foods to be found in this guide.

—Lack of regular exercise

Exercise is important for building and maintaining bone mass for all ages. Make sure you exercise at least thirty minutes four to five times a week. Weight-bearing exercises, such as walking, jogging, aerobics, jumping rope, stair climbing, and dancing, stimulate bone growth. Strength training also helps to keep bones strong. Be sure to include both types of exercise in your bone-boosting program.

—Certain medical problems

There are some illnesses that increase your risk of getting osteoporosis. They include rheumatoid arthritis, diabetes mellitus, emphysema, chronic bronchitis, and certain types of surgery on the stomach, as well as less common medical conditions. Ask your doctor if you are at increased risk and use the bone-boosting foods and other preventative measures to stay strong.

—Certain medications

Some medications, such as corticosteroids (for lung diseases, allergy, and arthritis), antacids with aluminum, cholesterol-lowering drugs, heparin, and some medications used to treat prostate cancer and endometriosis can increase bone loss. Ask your doctor if your medication increases your risk of osteoporosis. See if other bone-building medications can help counteract this problem.

—More than three cups of coffee or other caffeinated beverages daily

Although the studies are inconclusive, high amounts of caffeine might increase the amount of calcium lost through urine. A bone-saving idea is to limit caffeine intake to two or three cups a day. Add extra milk to these drinks, or use decaffeinated beverages.

—More than three alcoholic beverages daily

Alcohol causes appetite suppression, resulting in decreased intakes of essential bone-boosting foods. It also impairs the absorption of calcium in the intestine. If you do drink, do so in moderation (no more than two servings a day).

—Cigarette smoking

Smoking doubles your risk of osteoporosis, possibly by reducing the effectiveness of the body's estrogen. Also, smokers are often underweight (another risk factor for osteoporosis). Ask your doctor about a stop-smoking program or call the American Lung Association in your community.

—A diet high in animal protein

Studies show that when protein consumption increases, so does calcium excretion in the urine. Excess protein binds with calcium and flushes the mineral out of the body. Limit animal protein in your diet to two small servings a day, or replace meats with soy protein or lentils.

—A diet high in sodium

A high salt intake can increase your loss of bone. Reduce the high-sodium processed foods in your diet to prevent possible bone loss; eat more fresh fruits and vegetables.

—Depression

New research shows that women who suffer one or more episodes of major depression have lower bone density, although the exact causes are not known. Be sure to seek help if you are depressed, and ask your doctor if further treatment is needed.

RATE YOUR RISK

Risk Factors You *Can't* **Control**	**Risk Factors You** *Can* **Control**
___Family history	___Low calcium in the diet
___Race	___Having a bone density test
___Sex	___Lack of regular exercise
___Age	___Being underweight
___Menopause	___Heavy alcohol consumption
Certain diseases (see page 14)	___Smoking cigarettes
	___Diet high in sodium or protein
	___Certain medications (see page 14)
	___Excessive exercise in female athletes
	___No estrogen replacement after menopause
	___Excess caffeine consumption

SCORE OSTEOPOROSIS TEST

Take the following quiz to assess your risk for osteoporosis.

1. What is your current age? ___ years
   Take this number, multiply by 3, and enter result in this space.   ___Start

2. What is your race or ethnic group? (Check one)
   African-American ___ (Enter 0)
   Caucasian ___ Hispanic ___ Asian ___ (Enter 5)
   Native American ___ Other ___ (Enter 5)   ___

3. Have you ever been treated for or told you have rheuma-
   toid arthritis?
   Yes ___   No ___
   If yes, enter 4.   If no, enter 0.   ___

4. Since the age of 45, have you experienced a fracture (broken bone) at any of the following sites?

Hip   Yes ___   No ___   If yes, enter 4.   ___
Rib   Yes ___   No ___   If yes, enter 4.   ___
Wrist Yes ___   No ___   If yes, enter 4.   ___

5. Do you currently take or have you ever taken estrogen? (Examples include Premarin, Estrace, Estraderm, and Estratab.) If no, enter 1.   ___
Yes ___   No ___
Add score from questions 1 to 5.   ___**Subtotal**

6. What is your current weight? ___ pounds
Take your weight and subtract from the **subtotal** to receive your **score.**   ___**Score**
If your final score is 6 or greater, you should be evaluated further for osteoporosis. Talk to your doctor.

Staying Fracture-free

After assessing the stages and risk factors of osteoporosis, your goal should be to stay at the stage at which the disease can be controlled. This can keep you fracture-free for your entire lifetime. Start today to prevent osteoporosis by thinking B.O.N.E.S.

- **B**oost your intake of foods that promote bone strength.

- **O**btain a bone density test from your physician.

- **N**ote the risk factors over which you have control, and make plans to change them.

- **E**xercise regularly with weight-bearing and strength-training activities.

- **S**upplement your bone-boosting plan with bone-building medications or estrogen, if warranted.

The Importance of Calcium

Calcium is the key to preventing osteoporosis. We lose a certain amount every day and must replace it through dietary measures and calcium supplements.

Studies reveal that only 10 percent of all women get adequate amounts of calcium each day. The **Bone-Boosting Requirement (BBR)** needed for osteoporosis prevention varies from *800 milligrams* a day for a preschooler to *1,500 milligrams* a day for older children, teenage girls, pregnant women, postmenopausal women not taking estrogen, and men and women sixty-five and older. The average adult between ages twenty-five and sixty-five needs at least *1,000–1,500 milligrams* per day.

More than one-third of all American households supplement their diets with calcium. Included in this statistic are the more than 50 percent of pregnant women who use calcium supplements. Yet depending on the brand, you may be getting more than you bargained for. Recent findings from the **Natural Resources Defense Council** revealed that many calcium supplements exceed the standard safe lead level of .75 micrograms of lead per 1,000 milligrams of product (United States Pharmacopoeia). Lead is linked to high blood pressure, kidney problems, heart disease, and cancer. For small children and fetuses, lead can damage the central nervous system.

To stay on the safe side, try to get natural calcium through the bone-boosting foods in this book. If you use calcium supplementation, be sure to ask your doctor or pharmacist about a brand that is low in lead. When taking calcium supplements, think B.O.N.E.S. for best absorption:

- **B**e sure to take *no more* than 500 mg of supplemental calcium at one time.

- **O**nly take supplements with food for best absorption.

- **N**ever take supplements with iron, as calcium binds with iron and limits absorption.

- **E**xtra calcium taken before bedtime will give a bone-building boost during sleep.

- **S**pace supplements throughout the day to get the most benefit.

Another reason calcium-rich foods are the best source of calcium to keep bones strong is that foods offer myriad beneficial nutrients that supplements don't. A study in the *American Journal of Nutrition* reported on two groups of postmenopausal women who added to their diets either dry milk powder or calcium tablets. While both groups boosted calcium intake, because of milk's other nutrients, the women taking milk powder significantly boosted their intake of bone-boosting magnesium and zinc. Those taking calcium supplements did not.

BONE-BOOSTING REQUIREMENTS (BBR)

Children and Young Adults	Amount Per Day
0–12 months	210–270 mg
1–3 years	500 mg
4–8 years	800 mg
9–18 years	1,300–1,500 mg

Adult Women	
Pregnant and Lactating	1,000–1,300 mg
19–50 (premenopausal)	1,000 mg
51–64 (without estrogen)	1,500 mg
51–64 (with estrogen)	1,200 mg
65+ (with or without estrogen)	1,500 mg

Adult Men	
19–64	1,000 mg
65+	1,500 mg

Other Bone-Building Nutrients

While research on osteoporosis continues to point to a diet high in calcium as vital for bone strength, scientists have also identified the following bone-building nutrients to keep bones strong and help you stay fracture-free:

● **Vitamin A**—a *bone booster* necessary for normal bone growth and development. The **BBR** is 6,000 international units.

● **Vitamin C**—a *bone booster* necessary for the synthesis of collagen, a major component of bone. The **BBR** is 500 to 1,000 milligrams a day.

● **Vitamin D**—a *bone booster* that helps keep the right level of calcium and phosphorus in the bloodstream. When the body is low in vitamin D, the blood levels of calcium drop. While vitamin D is found in foods, most of this vitamin comes from sunshine. Going out-of-doors for fifteen to twenty minutes daily is a great way to boost vitamin D in the body. Yet, there are certain factors that hinder absorption, such as:

● wearing sunscreen out-of-doors
● aging
● working in an office during daytime hours
● getting sunshine through windowpane glass
● change of seasons
● latitude
● time of day

When the blood levels of calcium and phosphorus drop, where does the body turn for more of these minerals? You guessed it—your bones.

New research from Tufts University suggests that postmenopausal women need 400 international units a day of vitamin D for protection against osteoporosis. Research at Boston University reveals that osteoarthritis of the knee, a common problem associated with aging, progresses more slowly in seniors who consume at least 386 international units a day, compared with those who consumed the RDA (200 international units). These studies demonstrate that many older adults would benefit from supplementation. The **BBR is** 400 to 800 international units.

● **Vitamin K**—a newly identified *bone booster!* Research shows that vitamin K is essential in promoting the laying down of calcium and preventing osteoporosis. The **BBR** is 200 micrograms (mcg) for men and women.

● **Boron**—a *bone booster* that may increase estrogen levels in the blood and help women who take estrogen replacement therapy (ERT) to retain calcium and magnesium. You should get your **BBR** of 3 milligrams a day through a diet high in fresh fruits and vegetables.

● **Fluoride**—a *bone booster* that accumulates in new bone formation sites, resulting in a net gain in bone mass. The **BBR** is 1.5 to 4 milligrams.

● **Magnesium**—a *bone booster* that regulates active calcium transport and helps to prevent fractures. Sixty percent of dietary magnesium is stored in the bone. The **BBR** is 500 to 700 milligrams per day.

● **Manganese**—a *bone booster* and antioxidant involved in bone and connective tissue development. Some researchers feel that this trace mineral may be as important as calcium in building bone! The **BBR** is between 20 and 25 milligrams daily.

● **Phosphorus**—a *bone booster* that works side by side with calcium to build strong bones and teeth. In fact, approximately 85 percent of the phosphorous in the body is found in the bones. The **BBR** is 1,000 milligrams.

● **Zinc**—a *bone booster* important in the normal bone growth of children. It is part of the structure of bones, and is necessary for bones to rebuild. The **BBR** is 25 milligrams daily.

Supplement, Not *Substitute*

The recommended dietary allowances (RDAs) are the levels of nutrients thought to be adequate to meet the known nutrient needs of most healthy people. While the RDAs will help to prevent deficiency-related diseases such as beriberi or scurvy, there is groundbreaking scientific evidence that indicates certain nutrients should be ingested for disease prevention. In other words, the RDAs have not kept up with the medical breakthroughs.

Choosing a variety of healthful foods from this book will ensure that you are getting the proper nutrients needed to prevent osteoporosis. Of course, if your eating habits are poor, you may need supplementation with a multiple vitamin. Talk with a registered, licensed dietitian about your specific needs.

A New Superstar

Soybeans have played an essential role in Asian cultures for centuries. Heart disease, breast cancer, prostate cancer, and osteoporosis rates for Asian men and women are much lower than for Americans. Japanese women have half the rate of hip fracture of American women. Scientists attribute this to the high levels of phytoestrogens (plant estrogens) from eating a diet rich in soy.

The special isoflavones are compounds found in soy that are converted into phytoestrogens in the body. These plant ingredients mimic the hormone estrogen, but without the harmful side effects. Isoflavones appear to relieve menopausal symptoms that frequently occur because of plummeting estrogen levels during menopause. New studies have found that postmenopausal women with high concentrations of soy in their diet have stronger bones. These results indicate significant increases in both bone mineral content and bone density in the lumbar spine for women with a high soy diet. Not only is bone density increased with soy, but bone quality is improved as well. Studies show that soy protein isolate can also effectively prevent the ovarian-hormone-deficiency-associated rise in serum cholesterol.

Over the past decade, more than 2,000 new soy products have been introduced to American consumers, including meatless pepperoni, salami, hot dogs, bacon, puddings, and dairy alternatives. Calcium-rich soy foods include calcium-set tofu, fortified soy milk, textured vegetable protein, and soy nuts. While there is no set amount of isoflavones thought to help build bones, many researchers feel that one serving of soy a day can be helpful.

What Equals One Serving of Soy?

1 cup (8 ounces) soy milk
½ cup (2 to 3 ounces) tofu
½ cup rehydrated textured vegetable protein (TVP)

½ cup green soybeans
3-ounce soy protein concentrate burger

Bone-Boosting Superstars

Calcium Superstars

Blackstrap molasses
Calcium-fortified foods
Dairy products (such as milk, cheese, creamed cheese, yogurt, ice cream, and cottage cheese)
Dried figs
Greens, mustard and turnip

Okra
Orange
Salmon (canned with bones)
Sardines (canned with bones)
Tofu (processed with calcium sulfate)

Vitamin A Superstars

Apricot
Cantaloupe
Carrot
Greens, turnip
Kale
Liver, beef, chicken, and pork

Mango
Spinach
Sweet potato
Vitamin A–fortified foods

Vitamin C Superstars

Broccoli

Grapefruit

Guava

Kohlrabi

Mango

Orange

Papaya

Peppers, red and green

Strawberries

Vitamin C–fortified foods

Vitamin D Superstars

Dairy products

Eggs and egg substitutes

Herring

Liver, beef, chicken, and
  pork

Margarine

Mackerel

Salmon

Sardines

Tuna

Vitamin D–fortified foods

Vitamin K Superstars

Asparagus

Broccoli, raw

Dairy products

Eggs

Greens, collard, mustard,
  and turnip

Lentils

Liver, beef, chicken, and
  pork

Soybeans

Spinach, raw

Whole wheat products

Boron Superstars

Beans, dried

Fruit, fresh and dried

Greens, leafy

Nuts

Peas, dried

Seeds

Vegetables

Fluoride Superstars

Anchovies, with bones

Fluoridated drinking water

Milk

Salmon, with bones

Sardines, with bones

Seaweed

Tea, especially if made with
  fluoridated water

Vegetables grown in soil
  high in fluoride

Magnesium Superstars

Avocado

Banana

Dairy products

Legumes

Nuts

Parsnips

Seafood

Soybeans

Spinach

Whole grains

Manganese Superstars

Eggs

Green leafy vegetables

Lentils

Meat

Nuts

Seeds

Strawberries

Sweet potatoes

Tea

Whole grains

Phosphorus Superstars

Cheddar cheese

Eggs

Fish

Grains

Legumes

Meat

Milk

Nuts

Poultry

Tofu

Zinc Superstars

Almonds

Black-eyed peas

Crab

Meat

Milk

Peanut butter

Seafood

Sunflower seeds

Tofu

Wheat germ

Getting Started

Some bone-boosting vitamins and minerals are easy to get through a variety of foods. Because the Bone-Boosting Requirement (BBR) is low for vitamin K, boron, fluoride, and manganese, look through the Superstar lists on pages 23 to 25 to make sure you are on track. For example, a small serving of broccoli, brussels sprouts, collards, kale, or spinach gives you a day's worth of vitamin K. You can get ample vitamin D through sun exposure of fifteen to twenty minutes each day and by drinking some vitamin D–fortified milk.

Other bone-boosting foods containing such nutrients as vitamins A and C, calcium, magnesium, phosphorus, and zinc are not always included in your daily meal plan. If your diet is low in these nutrients, consider adding these, using the extensive list of foods in your **Bone-Boosting Guide.**

In the listing, you will find a wide variety of foods and beverages with their nutrient values given for commonly consumed portion sizes. Look at the suggested Bone-Boosting Requirements (BBR) on pages 19 to 21. Then using the listing of foods, make sure that you are eating the suggested requirements for these key nutrients. Foods that have small amounts of nutrients across the board should be eaten sparingly.

By combining favorite foods, you can increase their bone-boosting benefit. For example, a plain bagel is very low in the essential vitamins and minerals needed for strong bones. If you spread 1 ounce of low-fat cream cheese on top, you have boosted your vitamin A, calcium, phosphorus, and zinc intake for the day. Top the same plain bagel with two slices of low-fat American cheese, and you have met almost one-third of your daily calcium requirement, as well as having boosted your intake of vitamin A, phosphorus, and zinc. Add one glass of calcium-enriched orange or apple juice to boost vitamin C and calcium, and complement your meal with a spinach salad, high in bone-boosting magnesium and vitamins A and K.

Because it takes about 21 days to establish a habit such as an eating pattern, use the 21-Day Bone-Boosting Diary at the end of the book to record the foods eaten, the actual amounts, and the associated nutrients.

Super Bone Boosters

While most of the recipes presented in this book are low in fat, some may be higher than the 30 percent fat calories recommended to help you maintain a low-fat diet. Remember: Fruits and vegetables have little or no fat, yet vital bone-boosting foods like low-fat cheese may have 50 percent fat calories. To keep bones strong and to stay at a normal weight, learn to balance high- and low-fat foods over the course of the day and week. You can do this by adding fat-free fruits, vegetables, pastas, and grain products to complement your recipe.

Most people take in a large percentage of calories each day in refined, processed, low-fat or fat-free products, such as cookies and chips. While these may be low-fat, remember that *what you eat is more important that what you leave out.* We want you to focus on eating natural foods—foods high in bone-boosting vitamins and minerals that are listed in this counter and used in the 102 recipes.

Read the Label

To see if a food is high, moderate or low in fat, it is important to read the label. Package labels include the ingredients, the calories, the fat content, nutrients, the sodium and fiber content, and much more for the consumer's information (see sample label).

Sample Label

Kraft Natural Finely Shredded Parmesan Cheese

Ingredients: Part-skim milk, cheese culture, salt, enzymes, aged over 10 months.

Nutrition Facts

Serving size 2 tsp (5g)
Servings per container 17
Amount Per Serving
Calories 20
Calories from Fat 10

	% Daily Value*
Total Fat 1.5 g	2%
Saturated Fat 1 g	5%
Cholesterol less than 5 mg	1%

Sodium 75 mg	3%
Total Carbohydrate 0g	0%
Dietary Fiber 0g	0%
Sugars	0%
Protein 2g	
Vitamin A	0%
Calcium	4%
Vitamin C	0%
Iron	0%

*Percent Daily Values are based on a 2,000-calorie diet. Your daily values may be higher or lower depending on your calorie needs.

High or Low Fat?

After reading the label, you can figure out the fat content by using the following formula:

1 gram fat = 9 calories
If the serving has 2 grams of fat, then
$2 \times 9 = 18$ calories from fat
If the total calories for a serving are 100, then:
$18/100 = 18\%$ of calories from fat

Labels Can Be Confusing

- *Low-fat* means a product has no more than 3 grams of fat per serving.
- **Low saturated fat** means it has no more than 1 gram of saturated fat per serving.
- **Reduced fat** means the product has at least 25 percent less fat per serving than the traditional item.
- **Light** means the product has ½ the fat or ⅓ the calories of its regular counterpart.
- **Fat-free** has .5 gram of fat or less per serving.

Feed Those Bones!

Making the right choices in what we eat is a major concern for most of us. Food Marketing Institute (FMI) research shows that more than 70 percent of all shoppers think their diets could be more healthful. The American Dietetic Association (ADA) reports that 60 percent of all consumers are seeking guidelines on choosing healthful foods.

Whether you are a vegetarian or a meat-eater who wants to reduce—not eliminate—the amount of meat in your diet, we know that the time is right to rewrite your favorite recipes. Let the following Bone-Boosting Recipes start you on the right track to staying strong your entire lifetime.

Section Two

BONE-BOOSTING VITAMINS AND MINERALS

BEVERAGES	VIT A (IU)	VIT C (mg)	CAL (mg)	MAG (mg)	PHOS (mg)	ZINC (mg)
Alcoholic						
Beer, light (12 oz.)	0	0	18	18	43	0.11
Beer, regular (12 oz.)	0	0	18	21	43	0.07
Bloody Mary (5 oz.)	508	20	10	12	21	0.13
Daiquiri (2 oz.)	2	1	2	1	4	0.04
Screwdriver (7 oz.)	134	66	15	17	30	0.09
Tom Collins (7.5 oz.)	2	4	9	2	2	0.18
Wine, table, red (3.5 oz.)	0	0	8	13	14	0.09
Wine, table, white (3.5 oz.)	0	0	9	10	14	0.07
Nonalcoholic						
Carbonated						
Club soda (12 oz.)	0	0	18	4	0	0.36
Cola (12 oz.)	0	0	11	4	44	0.04
Cola, with aspartame (12 oz.)	0	0	14	4	32	0.28
Ginger ale (12 oz.)	0	0	11	4	0	0.18
Lemon-lime soda	0	0	7	4	0	0.18
Orange (12 oz.)	0	0	19	4	4	0.37
Root beer (12 oz.)	0	0	19	4	0	0.26
Tonic water (12 oz.)	0	0	4	0	0	0.37

Noncarbonated	VIT A (IU)	VIT C (mg)	CAL (mg)	MAG (mg)	PHOS (mg)	ZINC (mg)
Carob-flavor beverage mix, powder, prepared with milk (1 cup)	307	2	292	33	228	0.92
Chocolate-flavor beverage mix, powder, prepared with milk (1 cup)	311	2	301	53	255	1.28
Cocoa mix, with aspartame, powder, with added calcium, phosphorous, Swiss Miss, 1 envelope (.53 oz.)	240	0	216	31	245	0.52
Cocoa mix, with aspartame, powder, with added calcium, phosphorous, 1 packet (.675 oz.)	306	0	275	40	311	0.66
Cocoa mix, Nestlé, Carnation Hot Cocoa Mix with Marshmallows (28.0 g)	0	0	41	16	58	0.20
Cocoa mix, Nestlé, Carnation No Sugar Added Hot Cocoa Mix (15.0 g)	0	0	123	27	135	0.60
Cocoa mix, Nestlé, Carnation Rich Chocolate Hot Cocoa Mix (28.0 g)	0	0	40	27	71	0.36
Coffee, instant, decaffeinated, powder, prepared with water (6 oz.)	0	0	5	7	5	0.05

	VIT A (IU)	VIT C (mg)	CAL (mg)	MAG (mg)	PHOS (mg)	ZINC (mg)
Coffee, instant, regular, prepared with water (6 oz.)	0	0	5	7	5	0.05
Coffee, brewed, prepared with water (1 cup)	0	0	5	12	2	0.05
Fruit drink, frozen, prepared, McClain Citrus (100% vitamin C)						
Apple Melon (1 cup)	*	60	*	*	*	*
Kiwi Raspberry (1 cup)	*	60	*	*	*	*
Strawberry Lemon (1 cup)	*	60	*	*	*	*
Wild Berry Punch (1 cup)	*	60	*	*	*	*
Fruit punch drink, canned (1 cup)	35	73	20	5	2	0.30
Fruit punch-flavored drink, powder, prepared with water (1 cup)	0	31	42	3	52	0.08
Fruit punch drink, frozen concentrate, prepared with water (1 cup)	27	108	10	5	2	0.10
Gelatin, drink, orange-flavor, powder, prepared (1 packet)	0	50	3	1	0	0.03
Lemonade-flavor drink, powder, prepared with water (1 cup)	0	34	29	3	3	0.08
Lemonade, frozen concentrate, pink, prepared with water (1 cup)	5	10	7	5	5	0.10
Lemonade, with aspartame, powder, prepared with water (1 cup)	0	6	50	2	24	0.07

	VIT A (IU)	VIT C (mg)	CAL (mg)	MAG (mg)	PHOS (mg)	ZINC (mg)
Lemonade, powder, prepared with water (1 cup)	0	8	71	3	34	0.11
Malt beverage (1 cup)	5	1	12	17	52	0.05
Milk, chocolate beverage, hot cocoa, homemade (1 cup)	515	3	315	70	293	1.48
Nautilus Essentials, Soy and Milk Protein Isolate (1 packet)	5000	90	500	105	350	4.4
Nautilus Pro Drink, Milk Protein Isolate (1 packet)	2500	90	600	190	500	8
Nutri Joint, Knox unflavored gelatin drink mix, dietary supplement (1 scoop)	*	60	150	*	*	*
Orange drink, breakfast type with juice and pulp, frozen, concentrate, prepared with water (8 oz.)	15	138	293	28	83	0.13
Orange drink, breakfast type, powder, prepared with water (1 cup)	1835	121	62	2	37	0.10
Rice Beverage, Imagine Food Rice Dream, canned (1 cup)	5	1	20	10	34	0.25
Smoothie Mix, Fountain of Youth, vanilla yogurt and protein mix, NV/Nu Vigor, dry (1.62 oz.)	5000	60	1000	*	300	13
Strawberry-flavor beverage mix, powder, prepared with milk (1 cup)	309	2	293	32	229	0.93

	VIT A (IU)	VIT C (mg)	CAL (mg)	MAG (mg)	PHOS (mg)	ZINC (mg)
Tea, brewed, prepared with tap water (1 cup)	0	0	0	7	2	0.05
Tea, instant, unsweetened, powder, prepared (1 cup)	0	0	5	5	2	0.07
Tea, instant, unsweetened, lemon-flavored powder, prepared (1 cup)	0	0	5	5	2	0.07
Tea, herb, other than chamomile, brewed (1 cup)	0	0	4	2	0	0.07
Tea, herb, chamomile, brewed (1 cup)	47	0	5	2	0	0.10
Water, bottled, Perrier, unflavored (1 cup)	0	0	33	0	0	0.00
Water, municipal (1 cup)	0	0	5	2	0	0.07

BREADS, FLOUR, AND GRAINS

Breads

Assorted

	VIT A (IU)	VIT C (mg)	CAL (mg)	MAG (mg)	PHOS (mg)	ZINC (mg)
Banana, prepared (1 slice)	278	1	13	8	35	0.21
Boston brown, canned (1 slice)	39	0	32	28	50	0.23
Cornbread						
Dry mix (1 oz.)	33	0	16	7	139	0.16
Prepared with 2% milk (1 piece)	180	0	162	16	110	0.39
Prepared with whole milk (1 piece)	158	0	161	16	109	0.38
Cracked-wheat (1 slice)	0	0	11	13	38	0.31
Egg (1 slice)	30	0	37	8	42	0.32

	VIT A (IU)	VIT C (mg)	CAL (mg)	MAG (mg)	PHOS (mg)	ZINC (mg)
English muffin						
Mixed-grain (1 muffin)	4	0	129	29	98	0.64
Plain, enriched with calcium (1 muffin)	0	0	98	11	75	0.40
Plain, enriched, without calcium (1 muffin)	0	0	29	11	75	0.40
Raisin-cinnamon (1 muffin)	1	0	84	9	44	0.57
Whole-wheat (1 muffin)	0	0	175	47	186	1.06
French or Vienna (1 medium)	0	0	19	7	26	0.22
Indian fry-Navajo (5″ dia.)	0	0	210	14	141	0.45
Irish soda, prepared (1 slice)	116	0	49	14	68	0.34
Italian (1 large slice)	0	0	23	8	31	0.26
Mixed-grain (1 large slice)	0	0	29	17	56	0.41
Oat bran (1 slice)	2	0	20	9	32	0.29
Oat-bran, reduced-calorie (1 slice)	0	0	13	11	28	0.23
Oatmeal (1 slice)	4	0	18	10	34	0.28
Phyllo dough (1 sheet)	0	0	2	3	14	0.09
Pita, white, enriched (1 large)	0	0	52	16	58	0.50
Pita, whole-wheat (1 large pita)	0	0	10	44	115	0.97
Popovers (1 popover)	117	0	38	7	56	0.30
Protein, includes gluten (1 slice)	0	0	24	10	33	0.20
Pumpernickel (1 regular slice)	0	0	18	14	46	0.39
Pumpkin, prepared (1 slice)	3259	1	11	8	32	0.20

	VIT A (IU)	VIT C (mg)	CAL (mg)	MAG (mg)	PHOS (mg)	ZINC (mg)
Special formula, high-calcium, light (1 slice)	1	0	130	7	15	0.19
Special formula, high-calcium, dark (1 slice)	1	0	139	12	29	0.27
Raisin, enriched (1 slice)	1	0	17	7	28	0.19
Rye (1 slice)	1	0	23	13	40	0.37
Tortillas, ready to bake or fry, corn (1 med., 6″)	63	0	46	17	82	0.24
Wheat (1 slice)	0	0	26	12	38	0.26
Wheat, reduced-calorie (1 slice)	0	0	18	6	21	0.19
Wheat, whole (1 slice)	0	0	20	24	64	0.54
Wheat bran (1 slice)	0	0	27	29	67	0.49
Wheat germ (1 slice)	0	0	25	10	45	0.38
White, prepared with whole milk (1 slice)	19	0	21	7	44	0.24
White, reduced-calorie (1 slice)	1	0	22	6	31	0.31

Bagels

	VIT A (IU)	VIT C (mg)	CAL (mg)	MAG (mg)	PHOS (mg)	ZINC (mg)
Cinnamon raisin (4″ dia.)	65	1	17	19	69	0.67
Egg (4″ dia.)	97	1	12	22	75	0.69
Oat bran (4½″ dia.)	4	0	13	63	182	2.29
Plain (4″ dia.)	0	0	66	26	85	0.79
Roman Meal Original (1 piece)	0	0	*	*	*	*

Biscuits

	VIT A (IU)	VIT C (mg)	CAL (mg)	MAG (mg)	PHOS (mg)	ZINC (mg)
Buttermilk (4″ dia., prepared)	83	0	237	18	166	0.55
Plain (4″ dia., prepared)	83	0	237	18	166	0.55
Mixed grain, refrigerated dough (3″ dia.)	0	0	8	14	158	0.30

	VIT A (IU)	VIT C (mg)	CAL (mg)	MAG (mg)	PHOS (mg)	ZINC (mg)
Plain or buttermilk, refrigerated dough (2¼″ dia.)	0	0	4	4	98	0.10

Bread products

	VIT A (IU)	VIT C (mg)	CAL (mg)	MAG (mg)	PHOS (mg)	ZINC (mg)
Bread crumbs, dry, grated (1 cup)	1	0	245	50	159	1.32
Bread crumbs, seasoned (1 cup)	17	0	119	46	160	1.09
Bread sticks, plain (1 stick)	0	0	2	3	12	0.09
Bread stuffing, bread, dry (1 oz.)	0	0	28	11	40	0.26
Bread stuffing, cornbread, dry (1 oz.)	45	1	22	12	32	0.21
Croutons, plain (½ oz.)	0	0	11	4	16	0.13
Croutons, seasoned (½ oz.)	3	0	14	6	20	0.13

Breakfast breads

	VIT A (IU)	VIT C (mg)	CAL (mg)	MAG (mg)	PHOS (mg)	ZINC (mg)
French toast						
Prepared with 2% milk (1 slice)	315	0	65	11	76	0.44
Prepared with whole milk (1 slice)	298	0	64	11	76	0.44
Pancakes						
Frozen, with buttermilk (1 6″ pancake)	73	0	45	10	272	0.48
Plain, dry mix, including buttermilk (1 oz.)	19	0	68	10	184	0.20
Plain, dry mix, complete, prepared (1 6″ pancake)	25	0	97	15	257	0.30

	VIT A (IU)	VIT C (mg)	CAL (mg)	MAG (mg)	PHOS (mg)	ZINC (mg)
Pancakes, prepared from recipe						
Blueberry (6″)	153	2	159	12	116	0.42
Buckwheat (6″)	162	0	179	39	285	0.82
Buttermilk (6″)	81	0	121	12	107	0.48
Dry mix, prepared (7″)	68	0	93	15	252	0.35
Whole-wheat (6″)	292	1	323	59	481	1.34
Waffles						
Plain, dry mix, prepared (1 4″ square)	67	0	93	15	252	0.35
Plain, frozen, with buttermilk (1 4″ square)	448	0	77	7	140	0.19
Plain, prepared from recipe (7″)	171	0	191	14	143	0.51
Toaster pastry, fruit (1 Pop Tart)	501	0	14	9	58	0.34
Breakfast bar (1 bar)						
Chocolate chip (Carnation)	*	*	20	60	60	3
Chocolate crunch (Carnation)	*	*	20	60	60	3
Peanut butter w/ chocolate chips (Carnation)	*	*	20	60	60	3
Chocolate crunch, w/ chocolate chips (Carnation)	*	*	20	60	60	3

Crackers

	VIT A (IU)	VIT C (mg)	CAL (mg)	MAG (mg)	PHOS (mg)	ZINC (mg)
Cheese (1 Goldfish)	1	0	1	0	1	0.01
Cheese (1 Twig)	3	0	3	1	4	0.02
Cheese, low-sodium (1 Goldfish)	1	0	1	0	1	0.01
Cheese, Cheez-It (1 cup)	100	0	94	22	135	0.70

	VIT A (IU)	VIT C (mg)	CAL (mg)	MAG (mg)	PHOS (mg)	ZINC (mg)
Flatbread (1 cracker)	0	0	2	5	16	0.14
Matzo						
Egg (1 cracker)	12	0	11	7	45	0.21
Plain (1 cracker)	0	0	4	7	25	0.19
Whole-wheat (1 cracker)	0	0	7	38	86	0.09
Whole-wheat, low-salt (1 cracker)	0	0	2	4	12	0.09
Melba Toast (1 cracker)	0	0	3	2	6	0.06
Melba Toast, wheat (1 cracker)	0	0	2	3	8	0.08
Milk (1 cracker)	4	0	19	2	33	0.07
Oyster (1 cracker)	0	0	7	2	6	0.05
Oyster (1 cup)	0	0	54	12	47	0.35
Rye, crispbread (1 cracker)	0	0	3	8	27	0.24
Rye, cheese filling (1 cracker)	1	0	16	3	24	0.05
Saltines, fat-free, low sodium (3 crackers)	0	0	3	4	17	0.14
Saltines, soda (1 cracker)	0	0	7	2	6	0.05
Sandwich, cheese filling (1 sandwich)	2	0	18	3	28	0.04
Sandwich, with peanut butter (1 sandwich)	0	0	7	4	17	0.07
Sandwich, cheese, with peanut butter (1 sandwich)	22	0	6	4	23	0.08
Sandwich, wheat, with cheese (1 cracker)	5	0	14	4	27	0.06
Wafer (1 cracker)	0	0	8	20	67	0.60
Wheat crackers						
Euphrates (1 cracker)	0	0	2	32	9	0.06
Harvest (1 cracker)	0	0	1	2	7	0.05
Ritz (1 cracker)	0	0	1	2	7	0.05

	VIT A (IU)	VIT C (mg)	CAL (mg)	MAG (mg)	PHOS (mg)	ZINC (mg)
Wheat Thins (1 cracker)	0	0	1	2	7	0.05
Triscuits (1 cracker)	0	0	0	*	100	*
Whole-wheat (1 cracker)	0	0	7	38	86	0.09

Croissants

	VIT A (IU)	VIT C (mg)	CAL (mg)	MAG (mg)	PHOS (mg)	ZINC (mg)
Apple (1 med.)	154	0	17	7	33	0.59
Butter (1 med.)	307	0	21	9	60	0.43
Cheese (1 med.)	346	0	30	14	74	0.54

Muffins, prepared with 2% milk

	VIT A (IU)	VIT C (mg)	CAL (mg)	MAG (mg)	PHOS (mg)	ZINC (mg)
Blueberry (1 muffin)	80	1	108	9	83	0.31
Corn (1 muffin)	137	0	148	13	101	0.35
Oat bran (1 muffin)	10	0	36	90	214	1.05
Plain (1 muffin)	80	0	114	10	87	0.32
Wheat bran (1 muffin)	478	5	107	45	163	1.57

Muffins, prepared with whole milk

	VIT A (IU)	VIT C (mg)	CAL (mg)	MAG (mg)	PHOS (mg)	ZINC (mg)
Blueberry (1 muffin)	63	1	107	9	82	0.31
Corn (1 muffin)	117	0	147	13	100	0.35
Plain (1 muffin)	61	0	113	9	87	0.32
Wheat bran (1 muffin)	459	5	106	45	162	1.57
Cinnamon, refrigerated dough (1 roll)	0	0	10	4	104	0.10
Egg (1 roll)	26	0	21	9	35	0.32
French (1 roll)	2	0	35	8	32	0.29
Oat bran (1 roll)	3	0	28	10	34	0.28
Plain (1 roll)	0	0	30	24	64	0.57
Plain, prepared with 2% milk (1 roll)	118	0	21	7	44	0.25
Plain, prepared with whole milk (1 roll)	108	0	21	7	44	0.25
Sweet rolls, prepared with raisins (1 roll)	233	0	36	16	63	0.38

	VIT A (IU)	VIT C (mg)	CAL (mg)	MAG (mg)	PHOS (mg)	ZINC (mg)
Sweet rolls, prepared with cheese (1 roll)	135	0	78	13	65	0.42
Hamburger (1 roll)	0	0	60	9	38	0.27
Hamburger, mixed-grain (1 roll)	0	0	41	21	52	0.46
Hard (1 roll)	0	0	54	15	57	0.54
Hot dog (1 roll)	0	0	60	9	38	0.27
Hot dog, mixed-grain (1 roll)	0	0	41	21	52	0.46
Plain (1 roll)	129	1	43	10	46	0.35
Soft (1 roll)	0	0	30	24	63	0.57
Wheat (1 roll)	0	0	50	12	33	0.29
Whole-wheat, dinner roll (1 roll)	0	0	30	24	64	0.57
Whole-wheat, submarine (1 roll)	0	0	100	80	210	1.89

Flour

	VIT A (IU)	VIT C (mg)	CAL (mg)	MAG (mg)	PHOS (mg)	ZINC (mg)
Acorn, full fat (1 oz.)	15	0	12	31	29	0.18
Amaranth (1 cup)	0	8	298	519	887	6.2
Arrowroot (1 cup)	0	0	51	4	14	0.09
Buckwheat, whole-groat (1 cup)	0	0	49	301	404	3.74
Carob (1 cup)	1	0	358	56	81	0.95
Corn, masa, enriched (1 cup)	0	0	161	125	254	2.02
Corn, whole-grain, yellow (1 cup)	549	0	8	109	318	2.02
Cottonseed, partially defatted (1 cup)	408	2	449	678	1501	10.99
Peanut, defatted (1 cup)	0	0	84	222	456	3.06
Peanut, low-fat (1 cup)	0	0	78	29	305	3.59
Pecan (1 oz.)	34	1	9	34	78	1.45
Potato (1 cup)	0	34	59	158	319	2.92
Rice, brown (1 cup)	0	0	17	177	533	3.87
Rice, white (1 cup)	0	0	16	55	155	1.26
Rice bran, crude (1 cup)	0	0	67	922	1979	7.13

	VIT A (IU)	VIT C (mg)	CAL (mg)	MAG (mg)	PHOS (mg)	ZINC (mg)
Rice bran, crude (1 cup)	0	0	67	922	1979	7.13
Rye, medium (1 cup)	0	0	25	77	211	2.03
Semolina, enriched (1 cup)	0	0	28	78	227	1.75
Sesame, low-fat (1 oz.)	18	0	42	96	215	2.84
Sesame, partially defatted (1 oz.)	20	0	43	103	230	0.03
Soy, defatted (1 cup)	40	0	241	290	674	2.46
Soy, low-fat (1 cup)	35	0	165	202	522	1.04
Sunflower seed, partially defatted (1 cup)	31	1	73	221	441	3.17
Triticale, whole grain (1 cup)	0	0	46	199	417	3.46
Wheat, white, all-purpose, enriched (1 cup)	0	0	19	28	135	0.88
Wheat, white, all-purpose, enriched, calcium-fortified (1 cup)	0	0	315	28	135	0.87
Wheat, white, cake, enriched (1 cup)	0	0	19	22	117	0.85
Wheat, white, enriched (1 cup)	0	0	21	34	133	1.17
Wheat, white, tortilla mix, enriched (1 cup)	0	0	228	23	233	0.71
Wheat, whole (1 cup)	0	0	41	166	415	3.52

Grains

	VIT A (IU)	VIT C (mg)	CAL (mg)	MAG (mg)	PHOS (mg)	ZINC (mg)
Almond meal, partially defatted, without added salt (1 oz.)	0	0	120	82	259	0.8
Amaranth, cereal grain (½ cup)	0	4	149	260	444	3.1
Amaranth, cereal grain (1 cup)	0	8	298	519	887	6.2

	VIT A (IU)	VIT C (mg)	CAL (mg)	MAG (mg)	PHOS (mg)	ZINC (mg)
Barley (½ cup)	20.5	0	31	123	243	2.55
Barley (1 cup)	41	0	61	245	486	5.1
Barley, pearled, raw (½ cup)	22	0	29	79	221	2.13
Barley, pearled, raw (1 cup)	44	0	58	158	442	4.26
Bran						
Corn, crude (1 cup)	54	0	32	49	55	1.19
Oat, raw (1 cup)	0	0	55	221	670	2.92
Rice, crude (1 cup)	0	0	67	922	1979	7.13
Wheat, crude (1 cup)	0	0	42	354	588	4.22
Buckwheat groats, roasted, dry (1 cup)	0	0	28	362	523	3.7
Bulgar, cooked (½ cup)	0	0	18	58	73	1.04
Cornmeal						
Degermed, enriched, yellow (1 cup)	570	0	7	55	116	0.99
Self-rising, degermed, yellow (1 cup)	570	0	483	68	860	1.38
Self-rising, plain, enriched, white (1 cup)	0	0	440	105	991	2.4
Self-rising, wheat flour added, enriched (1 cup)	0	0	508	91	1107	2.4
Couscous, cooked (½ cup)	0	0	14	14	39	0.46
Couscous, cooked (1 cup)	0	0	28	28	78	0.92
Millet, cooked (½ cup)	0	0	3.5	53	120	1.09
Millet, cooked (1 cup)	0	0	7	106	240	2.18
Quinoa (½ cup)	0	0	51	179	349	2.8
Quinoa (1 cup)	0	0	102	357	697	5.61
Rice						
Brown, long-grained, cooked (½ cup)	0	0	10	2	81	0.62

	VIT A (IU)	VIT C (mg)	CAL (mg)	MAG (mg)	PHOS (mg)	ZINC (mg)
Brown, long-grained, cooked (1 cup)	0	0	19	4	162	1.24
White, glutinous, cooked (1/2 cup)	0	0	8	9	34	0.39
White, glutinous, cooked (1 cup)	0	0	16	18	68	0.78
White, long-grain, parboiled, enriched (1/2 cup)	0	0	17	11	37	0.27
White, long-grain, parboiled, enriched (1 cup)	0	0	33	21	74	0.54
Wild, cooked (1/2 cup)	0	0	3	27	68	1.1
Wild, cooked (1 cup)	0	0	5	53	135	2.2
Sesame meal, partially defatted (1 cup)	19	0	43	98	219	2.9
Semolina, enriched (1 cup)	0	0	28	79	227	1.75
Soy meal, defatted, raw (1 cup)	48	0	297	373	855	6.17
Triticale (1 cup)	0	0	71	250	687	6.62
Wheat germ (1/4 cup)	32	0	14	84	325	4.64
Wheat germ (1/2 cup)	64	0	28	168	650	9.28

CANDIES

	VIT A (IU)	VIT C (mg)	CAL (mg)	MAG (mg)	PHOS (mg)	ZINC (mg)
Almond Joy, 1 bar (1.76 oz.)	7	0	40	33	70	0.40
Bar None, 1 bar (1.5 oz.)	57	0	62	31	86	0.53
Cadbury's Caramello, 1 bar (1.6 oz.)	148	1	89	19	72	0.43
Caramels, chocolate-flavor roll, 1 bar (2.25 oz.)	5	0	15	20	25	0.34
Chocolate, baking, unsweetened, 1 square (1 oz.)	28	0	21	88	118	1.14

	VIT A (IU)	VIT C (mg)	CAL (mg)	MAG (mg)	PHOS (mg)	ZINC (mg)
Chocolate, chips, semisweet, 60 pieces (1 oz.)	6	0	9	33	37	0.46
Chocolate, sweet, 1 bar (1.45 oz.)	8	0	10	46	60	0.62
Chocolate, with nuts, prepared, 1 piece (19.0 g)	38	0	10	9	18	0.14
Demet's Turtles, 1 piece (17.0 g)	28	0	27	9	34	0.25
Fudge						
Brown sugar, with nuts, prepared, 1 piece (14.0 g)	11	0	16	7	12	0.09
Chocolate, prepared, 1 piece (17.0 g)	32	0	7	4	10	0.07
Chocolate with nuts, prepared, 1 piece (19.0 g)	38	0	10	9	18	0.14
Vanilla with nuts, prepared, 1 piece (15.0 g)	30	0	7	4	11	0.08
Golden Almond, 1 bar (3 oz.)	125	0	279	94	230	1.45
Golden Almond Solitaires, 1 package (3 oz.)	43	0	305	100	255	1.56
Goobers Chocolate Covered Peanuts, 1 package (1.375 oz.)	0	0	50	46	115	0.85
Gumdrops, starch jelly pieces, 10 gummy worms (74.0 g)	0	0	2	1	1	0.00
Jelly beans, 10 small (11.0 g)	0	0	0	0	0	0.01
Krackel, 1 bar (1.65 oz.)	23	0	84	26	104	0.57
M & M's Milk Chocolate Mini-Baking Bits, 1 serving (14.2 g)	32	0	16	7	24	0.15

	VIT A (IU)	VIT C (mg)	CAL (mg)	MAG (mg)	PHOS (mg)	ZINC (mg)
M & M's Peanut Chocolate Candies, 1 package (1.67 oz.)	44	0	48	29	89	0.64
M & M's Plain Chocolate Candies, 1 package (1.69 oz.)	97	0	50	20	72	0.46
M & M's Semisweet Chocolate Mini- Baking Bits (1 tbsp.)	10	0	5	15	17	0.21
Milk chocolate candies, 1 bar (1.55 oz.)	81	0	84	26	95	0.61
Milk chocolate–coated peanuts, 10 pieces (40.0 g)	0	0	42	36	85	0.75
Mints, After Eight, 5 pieces (41.0 g)	8	0	9	19	23	0.24
Mounds, 1 package (1.9 oz.)	5	0	12	37	65	0.56
Mr. Goodbar, 1 bar (1.75 oz.)	20	0	56	48	140	0.90
Oh Henry! Bar, 1 bar (2 oz.)	27	0	62	35	103	0.70
Raisinets Chocolate Covered Raisins, 1 package (1.51 cup)	17	0	49	20	65	0.36
Reese's Peanut Butter Cups, 1 package (1.6 oz.)	30	0	35	38	108	0.63
Reese's Pieces Candy, 1 package (1.95 oz.)	11	0	73	46	127	0.61
Rolo Caramels in Milk Chocolate, 1 piece (3.0 g)	2	0	4	1	5	0.02
Skør Toffee Candy Bar, 1 bar (1.4 oz.)	112	0	45	14	60	0.30
Snickers Bar, 1 bar (2 oz.)	87	0	54	39	105	0.81

	VIT A (IU)	VIT C (mg)	CAL (mg)	MAG (mg)	PHOS (mg)	ZINC (mg)
Special Dark Sweet Chocolate Bar, Hershey, 1 bar (1.45 oz)	8	0	8	47	66	0.62
Symphony Milk Chocolate Bar, 1 bar (1.4 oz.)	28	0	94	22	100	0.45
Twix Caramel Cookie Bars, 1 package (2.06 oz.)	55	0	52	19	70	0.45
Twix Peanut Butter Cookie Bar, 1 package, 2 bars (1.89 oz.)	39	0	42	40	103	0.76
Twizzlers, Strawberry Candy (5 oz. package)	0	0	50	9	440	0.23
Yogurt, confectioner's coating candy (50 g edible portion)	18	0	100	6	88	0.37
York Peppermint Pattie, 1 large patty (43.0 g)	2	0	7	27	41	0.33

CEREALS

Hot, Measured, Uncooked

	VIT A (IU)	VIT C (mg)	CAL (mg)	MAG (mg)	PHOS (mg)	ZINC (mg)
Corn grits, instant, plain, Quaker (1 packet)	0	0	6	10	31	0.19
Corn grits, yellow, enriched, dry (1 tbsp.)	43	0	0	3	7	0.04
Cream of Rice (1/4 cup)	0	0	10	10	54	0.48
Cream of Rice (1/2 cup)	0	0	20	20	108	0.96
Cream of Wheat, mix'n eat, plain (1 packet)	1250	0	20	8	20	0.24
Cream of Wheat, instant (2 tbsp.)	0	0	32	8	24	0.22

	VIT A (IU)	VIT C (mg)	CAL (mg)	MAG (mg)	PHOS (mg)	ZINC (mg)
Cream of Wheat, regular (2 tbsp.)	0	0	30	6	24	0.18
Malt-O-Meal, plain (2 tbsp.)	0	0	3	3	15	0.10
Mother's Oat Bran (1/2 cup)	40	0	32	96	278	1.68
Oatmeal, MultiGrain, Quaker (1/2 cup)	3	0	14	46	138	1.28
Oatmeal, instant, Power Ranger, fruit punch flavor, Quaker (1 packet)	1273	0	176	35	121	0.80
Oatmeal, instant, Quaker, Apples and Cinnamon (1 packet)	1050	0	106	30	116	0.69
Oatmeal, instant, Quaker, Maple and Brown Sugar (1 packet)	1008	0	105	39	132	0.90
Roman Meal, plain (1/3 cup)	0	0	20	74	146	1.21
Wheatena (1/4 cup)	0	0	10	46	134	1.54

Ready to Eat

	VIT A (IU)	VIT C (mg)	CAL (mg)	MAG (mg)	PHOS (mg)	ZINC (mg)
All-Bran (1/2 cup)	750	15	106	129	294	3.75
All-Bran with extra fiber (1/2 cup)	866	17	116	120	287	4.32
Basic 4 (1 cup)	1250	15	310	40	232	3.75
Berry Berry Kix (3/4 cup)	750	15	66	6	37	3.75
Boo Berry (1 cup)	0	15	20	3	31	3.75
Bran, 100% (1 cup)	0	63	46	312	801	5.74
Bran Buds (1/3 cup)	750	15	20	83	166	6.45
Bran Chex (1 cup)	107	26	29	69	173	6.48
Bran Flakes, 40%, Ralston Purina (1 cup)	2160	26	23	118	273	2.04
Cap'n Crunch (3/4 cup)	36	0	5	10	29	3.75
Cheerios (1 cup)	1250	15	55	33	114	3.75

	VIT A (IU)	VIT C (mg)	CAL (mg)	MAG (mg)	PHOS (mg)	ZINC (mg)
Apple Cinnamon (¾ cup)	750	15	35	20	65	3.75
Honey Nut (1 cup)	750	15	20	29	103	3.75
Multigrain (1 cup)	750	15	57	30	114	3.75
Cinnamon Toast (¾ cup)	750	15	42	14	74	3.75
Clusters (1 cup)	0	9	72	52	153	1.05
Cocoa Krispies (¾ cup)	750	15	4	11	29	1.49
Cocoa Pebbles (1 cup)	1411	0	6	13	25	1.70
Cocoa Puffs (1 cup)	0	15	33	7	43	3.75
Common Sense (¾ cup)	750	0	15	48	153	3.75
Complete Bran Flakes (¾ cup)	1208	15	14	60	150	3.75
Corn Chex (1 cup)	146	15	3	4	11	0.10
Corn Flakes, Kellogg (1 cup)	700	14	1	3	11	0.17
Corn Flakes, Ralston Purina (1 cup)	95	0	2	3	10	0.06
Corn Pops (1 cup)	775	16	3	3	7	1.55
Count Chocula (1 cup)	0	15	29	9	41	3.75
Country Corn Flakes (1 cup)	750	15	53	7	39	3.75
Cracklin' Oat Bran (¾ cup)	842	17	25	77	187	1.65
Crispix (1 cup)	750	15	4	7	27	1.51
Crispy Wheaties 'N Raisins (1 cup)	1250	0	69	42	140	1.08
Crunchy Bran (¾ cup)	38	0	21	14	36	3.75
Fiber One (½ cup)	0	9	59	68	168	1.24
Frankenberry (1 cup)	0	15	25	3	28	3.75
Froot Loops (1 cup)	703	14	3	9	21	3.75
Frosted Bran (¾ cup)	726	15	9	38	92	3.63
Frosted Flakes (¾ cup)	775	16	1	3	8	0.16
Fruity Pebbles (1 cup)	1411	0	4	9	19	1.70
Golden Grahams (¾ cup)	750	15	14	9	36	3.75
Granola, homemade (1 cup)	45	2	99	217	564	4.95

	VIT A (IU)	VIT C (mg)	CAL (mg)	MAG (mg)	PHOS (mg)	ZINC (mg)
Granola, Low-Fat, Kellogg (½ cup)	842	0	23	47	135	4.24
Granola, Low-Fat with Raisins, Kellogg (⅔ cup)	688	0	24	46	127	3.47
Grape-Nuts (½ cup)	2403	0	5	37	137	1.20
Grape-Nuts Flakes (1 oz.)	1250	0	11	31	84	0.57
Healthy Choice Multi-Grain Flakes (1 cup)	500	0	9	29	86	1.50
Heartland Natural Cereal, Plain (1 cup)	64	1	75	147	416	3.04
Heartland Natural Cereal with Coconut (1 cup)	57	1	66	138	380	2.74
Heartland Natural Cereal with Raisins (1 cup)	63	1	66	141	377	2.83
Honey Bran (1 cup)	1543	19	16	46	132	0.90
Just Right (1 cup)	1250	0	14	34	106	0.88
Just Right Fruit & Nut (1 cup)	1146	0	0	33	109	1.05
Kaboom (1¼ cup)	750	15	50	19	88	3.75
King Vitaman (1½ cup)	1044	12	4	26	79	3.91
Life, Cinnamon (1 cup)	16	0	135	42	181	6.29
Life (¾ cup)	12	0	98	31	136	4.00
Maltex (¼ cup)	0	0	14	42	133	1.38
Mueslix Apple & Almond Crunch (¾ cup)	778	0	34	63	175	3.14
Mueslix Raisin & Almond Crunch, with Dates (⅔ cup)	200	0	20	47	133	3.74
Natural Bran Flakes, Post (1 cup)	2072	0	21	102	296	2.49
Natural Cereal, 100%, with Apple and Cinnamon, Quaker (1 oz.)	16	0	43	20	96	0.54

	VIT A (IU)	VIT C (mg)	CAL (mg)	MAG (mg)	PHOS (mg)	ZINC (mg)
Natural Cereal, 100%, with Oats and Honey, Quaker (½ cup)	3	0	46	50	149	1.15
Natural Cereal, 100% with Oats, Honey, and Raisins, Quaker (½ cup)	4	0	39	48	150	1.08
Natural Cereal, 100% with Raisins and Dates, Quaker (1 oz.)	16	0	41	32	90	0.54
Nature Valley, Cinnamon & Raisins Granola (¾ cup)	0	0	43	55	160	0.91
Nature Valley Low-Fat Fruit Granola (⅔ cup)	0	0	40	19	180	0.88
Nut & Honey Crunch (1¼ cup)	750	15	6	5	36	0.39
Nutri-Grain, Almond and Raisin (30 g)	0	0	102	8	113	2.4
Nutri-Grain, Wheat (¾ cup)	0	15	10	24	108	3.75
Nuttlettes (½ cup)	*	*	160	*	*	*
Oat Flakes, Post (1 cup)	2116	0	68	58	176	2.54
Oatmeal Crisp with Almonds (1 cup)	0	9	36	57	144	3.75
Oatmeal Squares, Quaker (1 cup)	563	7	36	70	186	4.22
Product 19 (1 cup)	750	60	3	12	40	15.00
Puffed Rice, Quaker (1 cup)	0	0	1	4	17	0.15
Puffed Wheat, Quaker (1¼ cup)	2	0	4	20	50	0.46
Raisin Bran, Kellogg (1 cup)	832	0	40	89	214	4.15
Raisin Bran, Post (1 cup)	2469	0	26	95	235	2.97
Raisin Bran, Ralston Purina (1 cup)	1852	2	27	85	248	1.67

	VIT A (IU)	VIT C (mg)	CAL (mg)	MAG (mg)	PHOS (mg)	ZINC (mg)
Raisin Nut Bran, General Mills (1 cup)	0	0	74	54	163	1.11
Raisin Squares, Kellogg (¾ cup)	0	0	19	48	160	1.54
Rice Chex (1 cup)	20	18	5	8	32	0.46
Rice Krispies (1¼ cup)	825	17	3	16	44	0.60
Rice Krispies, Apple-Cinnamon (¾ cup)	776	16	2	8	25	0.33
Rice Krispies Treats Cereal (¾ cup)	750	15	2	6	20	0.30
S'mores Grahams (¾ cup)	750	15	14	11	41	3.75
Shredded wheat, large biscuit (1 oblong biscuit)	0	0	10	43	91	0.63
Shredded wheat, small biscuit (1 cup)	0	0	9	33	88	0.82
Special K (1 cup)	750	15	5	18	51	3.75
Strawberry Squares (1 cup)	0	0	22	66	169	1.65
Sugar Frosted Flakes, Ralston (1 cup)	1675	20	4	3	10	0.82
Sun Country Granola, Raisin and Date (½ cup)	0	0	24	26	92	0.50
Super Sugar Crisp (1 cup)	1455	0	7	20	44	1.75
Team (1 cup)	1852	22	6	12	65	0.58
Toasted Brown Sugar Squares, Healthy Choice (1¼ cup)	509	0	19	59	194	1.54
Total (¾ cup)	1250	60	258	32	211	15.00
Total Corn Flakes (1⅓ cup)	1250	60	237	8	110	15.00
Total Raisin Bran (1 cup)	1250	0	238	45	259	14.00
Tripples (1 cup)	1250	15	41	7	35	3.75
Uncle Sam, Low-Sodium (1 cup)	*	1	40	*	*	*

	VIT A (IU)	VIT C (mg)	CAL (mg)	MAG (mg)	PHOS (mg)	ZINC (mg)
Wheat Chex (1 cup)	0	24	18	58	182	1.23
Wheat germ, toasted, plain (1 oz.)	0	2	13	91	325	4.72
Wheat germ, Kretchmer Honey Crunch (1⅔ tbsp.)	13	0	7	38	142	1.94
Wheaties (1 cup)	750	15	55	32	96	0.71

CHEESES

	VIT A (IU)	VIT C (mg)	CAL (mg)	MAG (mg)	PHOS (mg)	ZINC (mg)
American, pasteurized process, 1 slice (1 oz.)	343	0	175	6	211	0.85
Blue (1 oz.)	204	0	150	7	110	0.75
Brick (1 oz.)	307	0	191	7	128	0.74
Brie (1 oz.)	189	0	52	6	53	0.68
Camembert (1 oz.)	262	0	110	6	98	0.68
Caraway (1 oz.)	299	0	191	6	139	0.83
Cheddar (1 oz.)	300	0	205	8	145	0.88
Cheddar, low-fat (1 oz.)	66	0	118	5	137	0.52
Cheddar, low sodium (1 oz.)	297	0	200	8	137	0.88
Cheshire (1 oz.)	279	0	182	6	131	0.79
Colby (1 oz.)	293	0	194	7	129	0.87
Colby, low-fat (1 oz.)	66	0	118	5	137	0.52
Cottage cheese						
Calcium enriched, 1% fat (½ cup)	0	0	200	*	*	*
Creamed, large curd, not packed (1 cup)	367	0	135	12	297	0.83
Creamed, small curd, not packed (1 cup)	367	0	135	12	297	0.83
Creamed, with fruit, not packed (1 cup)	278	0	108	9	236	0.66
Lactose-reduced, 1% fat (½ cup)	0	0	100	*	*	*

	VIT A (IU)	VIT C (mg)	CAL (mg)	MAG (mg)	PHOS (mg)	ZINC (mg)
1% fat, not packed (1 cup)	84	0	138	12	302	0.86
2% fat, not packed (1 cup)	158	0	155	14	340	0.95
Uncreamed, dry, large or small curd, not packed (1 cup)	44	0	46	6	151	0.68
Cream cheese (1 oz.)	405	0	23	2	30	0.15
Cream cheese, fat-free (100 g)	930	0	185	14	434	0.88
Edam (1 oz.)	260	0	207	8	152	1.06
Feta (1 oz.)	127	0	140	5	96	0.82
Fontina (1 oz.)	333	0	156	4	98	0.99
Fondue, cheese (½ cup)	447	0	514	25	331	2.12
Gjetost (1 oz.)	316	0	113	20	126	0.32
Goat, hard type (1 oz.)	451	0	254	15	207	0.45
Goat, semisoft type (1 oz.)	378	0	85	8	106	0.19
Goat, soft (1 oz.)	378	0	40	4	73	0.26
Gouda (1 oz.)	183	0	198	8	155	1.11
Gruyère (1 oz.)	346	0	287	10	172	1.11
Limburger (1 oz.)	363	0	141	6	112	0.6
Monterey (1 oz.)	269	0	212	8	126	0.85
Mozzarella						
Part skim (1 oz.)	166	0	183	7	131	0.78
Part skim, low-moisture (1 oz.)	178	0	207	8	149	0.89
Whole milk (1 oz.)	225	0	147	5	105	0.63
Whole milk, low-moisture (1 oz.)	256	0	163	6	117	0.01
Muenster (1 oz.)	318	0	203	8	133	0.8
Neufchatel (1 oz.)	322	0	21	2	39	0.15
Parmesan						
Grated (1 oz.)	199	0	390	14	229	0.9
Grated (1 tbsp.)	35	0	69	3	40	0.16
Hard (1 oz.)	171	0	336	12	197	0.78
Lactose-Free, Parmesan Flavor, Grated Topping, Formagg (2 tbsp.)	0	0	60	*	*	*

	VIT A (IU)	VIT C (mg)	CAL (mg)	MAG (mg)	PHOS (mg)	ZINC (mg)
Pimento, pasteurized pimento (1 oz.)	358	1	174	6	211	0.85
Port du salut (1 oz.)	378	0	184	7	102	0.74
Provolone (1 oz.)	231	0	214	8	141	0.92
Queso anejo, Mexican (1 oz.)	63	0	193	8	126	0.83
Queso asadero, Mexican (1 oz.)	63	0	188	7	126	0.86
Ricotta, part-skim milk (1 oz.)	122	0	77	4	52	0.38
Ricotta, whole milk (1/2 cup)	608	0	257	14	196	1.44
Romano (1 oz.)	162	0	302	12	216	0.73
Roquefort (1 oz.)	297	0	188	8	111	0.59
Sauce, cheese, prepared (2 tbsp.)	182	0	93	6	69	0.39
Swiss, pasteurized (1 oz.)	229	0	219	8	216	1.02
Swiss, Reduced Fat, Sargento (1 slice)	500	*	300	*	*	*
Tilsit (1 oz.)	296	0	198	4	142	0.99

DESSERTS AND TOPPINGS

	VIT A (IU)	VIT C (mg)	CAL (mg)	MAG (mg)	PHOS (mg)	ZINC (mg)
Apple crisp, prepared (1/2 cup)	193	3	39	10	35	0.23
Brownies						
Commercially prepared (1 Little Debbie package twin)	42	0	18	19	62	0.44
Dry mix, prepared, 1 brownie (2″ square)	15	0	6	11	26	0.2
Dry mix, special dietary prepared, 1 brownie (2″ square)	0	0	3	1	11	0.03

	VIT A (IU)	VIT C (mg)	CAL (mg)	MAG (mg)	PHOS (mg)	ZINC (mg)
Prepared from recipe, 1 brownie (2″ square)	184	0	14	13	32	0.23

Cakes

	VIT A (IU)	VIT C (mg)	CAL (mg)	MAG (mg)	PHOS (mg)	ZINC (mg)
Angel food Commercially prepared (1 slice)	0	0	40	3	66	0.02
Dry mix, prepared (1 piece)	0	0	42	4	116	0.07
Prepared from recipe (1 piece)	0	0	3	5	13	0.07
Boston cream pie, prepared from recipe (1 piece)	180	0	93	16	91	0.44
Carrot, dry mix, pudding-type without frosting, 1 piece (1/12 of 9″ dia.)	790	2	77	5	123	0.22
Carrot, prepared from recipe with cream cheese frosting (1 piece)	3827	1	28	20	79	0.54
Cheesecake Commercially prepared (1 piece)	442	1	41	9	74	0.41
Plain, prepared from recipe with cherry topping (1 piece)	1275	1	61	10	101	0.57
Prepared from mix, no-bake type (1 piece)	362	1	170	19	232	0.46
Prepared from recipe (1 piece)	1354	1	74	10	123	0.7

	VIT A (IU)	VIT C (mg)	CAL (mg)	MAG (mg)	PHOS (mg)	ZINC (mg)
Chocolate, commercially prepared with chocolate frosting (1 piece)	61	0	28	22	78	0.16
Chocolate, dry mix, pudding-type, prepared without frosting (1 piece)	81	1	64	19	146	0.49
Coffee cake						
Cheese (1 piece)	178	0	45	11	75	0.45
Cinnamon with crumb topping (1 piece)	61	0	34	14	68	0.51
Fruit (1 piece)	70	0	23	9	59	0.33
Commercially prepared (1 piece)	34	0	14	7	23	0.12
Fruitcake, prepared from recipe (1 piece)	61	4	55	29	66	0.59
Pineapple upside-down, prepared from recipe (1/9 of 8" square)	291	1	138	15	94	0.36
Pound						
Commercially prepared, with butter (1 oz.)	172	0	10	3	39	0.13
Commercially prepared, fat-free (1 oz.)	27	0	12	3	41	0.09
Prepared from recipe, with butter (1/16 of loaf cake)	524	0	13	5	44	0.27
Shortcake, biscuit-type, prepared from recipe (1 cake, 3" dia.)	47	0	133	10	93	0.31

	VIT A (IU)	VIT C (mg)	CAL (mg)	MAG (mg)	PHOS (mg)	ZINC (mg)
Sponge, prepared from recipe, 1 piece (1/12 of 16 oz. cake)	163	0	27	6	63	0.37
White						
Prepared from recipe, with coconut frosting (1 piece)	43	0	101	13	78	0.37
Prepared from recipe, without frosting (1 piece)	41	0	96	9	69	0.24
Dry mix, pudding-type, without frosting (1 piece)	0	0	35	5	123	0.12
Yellow, dry mix, pudding-type, without frosting (1 piece)	80	0	57	5	133	0.26
Yellow, prepared from recipe, without frosting (1 piece)	95	0	99	8	80	0.31

Cookies

	VIT A (IU)	VIT C (mg)	CAL (mg)	MAG (mg)	PHOS (mg)	ZINC (mg)
Animal crackers (2 oz.)	0	0	25	10	65	0.37
Arrowroot (2 oz.)	0	0	25	10	65	0.37
Butter, commercially prepared, enriched (1 cookie)	30	0	2	1	5	0.02
Chocolate chip						
Chips Ahoy, Nabisco (1 cookie)	1	0	4	4	15	0.09
Chocolate Chunk Pecan, Pepperidge Farm (1 cookie)	1	0	3	4	13	0.08
Commercially prepared, regular, lower fat (1 cookie)	0	0	2	3	8	0.07

	VIT A (IU)	VIT C (mg)	CAL (mg)	MAG (mg)	PHOS (mg)	ZINC (mg)
Commercially prepared, soft, lower fat (1 cookie)	0	0	2	5	8	0.07
Refrigerated dough (1 med. cookie)	7	0	3	3	9	0.07
Rich 'n Chips, Pecan Chips, Keebler (1 large cookie)	1	0	4	4	15	0.09
Chocolate sandwich, with cream filling (1 cookie)	0	0	3	5	10	0.08
Chocolate sandwich, with extra cream (1 cookie)	0	0	3	4	12	0.09
Chocolate wafers (1 wafer)	1	0	2	3	8	0.07
Coconut macaroons, prepared from recipe (1 cookie)	0	0	2	5	10	0.17
Fig (1 cookie)	7	0	10	4	10	0.06
Fortune (1 cookie)	1	0	1	1	3	0.01
Fudge, cake-type (1 cookie)	0	0	7	7	17	0.17
Gingersnaps (1 cookie)	0	0	5	3	6	0.04
Graham crackers, plain or honey, includes cinnamon (2½″ square)	0	0	2	2	7	0.06
Ladyfingers, 1 anisette sponge (4″)	72	1	6	2	23	0.15
Ladyfingers, with lemon juice and rind (1 ladyfinger)	61	0	5	1	19	0.13
Marshmallow, chocolate-coated, includes marshmallow pie (1 pie)	1	1	18	14	38	0.25

	VIT A (IU)	VIT C (mg)	CAL (mg)	MAG (mg)	PHOS (mg)	ZINC (mg)
Molasses (1 cookie)	0	0	15	10	19	0.09
Oatmeal						
Commercially prepared, fat-free (1 cookie)	0	0	11	10	30	0.18
Commercially prepared, soft-type (1 cookie)	5	0	14	5	31	0.07
Prepared from recipe, with raisins (1 cookie)	96	0	15	6	24	0.13
Peanut butter, prepared from recipe (1 cookie)	120	0	8	8	23	0.16
Peanut butter, refrigerated dough (1 cookie)	6	0	13	5	32	0.09
Raisin, soft-type (1 cookie)	6	0	7	3	12	0.05
Shortbread, commercially prepared plain (1 med. cookie)	3	0	3	1	9	0.04
Shortbread, prepared from recipe, made with butter (1 med. cookie)	136	0	2	1	8	0.05
Sugar, prepared from recipe, made with butter, 1 cookie (3″ dia.)	125	0	10	2	13	0.06
Sugar, refrigerated dough, baked (1 cookie)	4	0	11	1	22	0.03
Tea biscuits (2 oz.)	0	0	25	10	65	0.37
Vanilla sandwich, cream filling (1 med. cookie)	0	0	3	1	8	0.04

	VIT A (IU)	VIT C (mg)	CAL (mg)	MAG (mg)	PHOS (mg)	ZINC (mg)
Vanilla wafers, lower fat (1 med. cookie)	2	0	2	1	4	0.01
Vanilla wafers, higher fat (1 med. cookie)	0	0	2	1	4	0.02

Custards

	VIT A (IU)	VIT C (mg)	CAL (mg)	MAG (mg)	PHOS (mg)	ZINC (mg)
Caramel, flan, dry mix, prepared with 2% milk (½ cup)	249	1	153	17	116	0.48
Caramel, flan, dry mix, prepared with whole milk (½ cup)	153	1	150	16	114	0.47
Caramel, flan, prepared from recipe (½ cup)	314	1	132	17	145	0.72
Egg custard						
Dry mix, prepared with 2% milk (½ cup)	295	1	197	27	176	0.71
Dry mix, prepared with whole milk (½ cup)	200	1	194	25	174	0.69
Dry mix, prepared from recipe, 1 piece (⅛ of 9″ dia.)	281	1	107	17	125	0.62

Doughnuts

	VIT A (IU)	VIT C (mg)	CAL (mg)	MAG (mg)	PHOS (mg)	ZINC (mg)
Cake-type						
Chocolate, sugared, glazed, 1 med. (approx. 3″ dia.)	37	0	90	14	68	0.24
Plain, unsugared, old-fashioned, 1 med. (3¼″ dia.)	27	0	21	9	126	0.26
Wheat, sugared or glazed, 1 med. (approx. 3″ dia.)	29	0	22	10	47	0.31
French crullers, glazed (3″ dia.)	7	0	11	5	50	0.12

	VIT A (IU)	VIT C (mg)	CAL (mg)	MAG (mg)	PHOS (mg)	ZINC (mg)
Yeast-leavened, cream filling 1 med. (3½" × 2½" oval)	25	0	21	17	65	0.68
Yeast-leavened, glazed, enriched, includes honey buns (1 bun)	27	0	34	17	73	0.6
Yeast-leavened, with jelly filling, 1 med. (3½" × 2½" oval)	26	1	21	17	72	0.64

Frostings

	VIT A (IU)	VIT C (mg)	CAL (mg)	MAG (mg)	PHOS (mg)	ZINC (mg)
Chocolate, creamy, prepared from recipe, with margarine (1/12 package)	219	0	9	13	24	0.2
Cream cheese–flavor, ready to eat (1/12 package)	146	0	1	1	1	0
Sour cream–flavor, ready-to-eat (1/12 package)	152	0	1	1	2	0
Vanilla, creamy, ready-to-eat (1/12 package)	284	0	1	0	15	0

Frozen Desserts

	VIT A (IU)	VIT C (mg)	CAL (mg)	MAG (mg)	PHOS (mg)	ZINC (mg)
Fruit and juice bars, 1 bar (3 fl. oz.)	27	9	5	4	6	0.05
Gelatins, dry mix, reduced-calorie, with aspartame (½ cup)	0	12	0	0	0	0
Ice cream, chocolate (½ cup)	275	1	72	19	71	0.38
Ice cream, chocolate (1 cup)	550	2	144	38	142	0.76

	VIT A (IU)	VIT C (mg)	CAL (mg)	MAG (mg)	PHOS (mg)	ZINC (mg)
Ice cream, French vanilla, soft-serve (1/2 cup)	464	1	113	10	100	0.45
Ice cream, French vanilla, soft-serve (1 cup)	928	2	226	20	200	0.9
Ice cream, strawberry (1/2 cup)	211	5	79	9	66	0.22
Ice cream, strawberry (1 cup)	422	10	158	18	132	0.44
Ice cream, vanilla (1/2 cup)	270	0	85	9	69	0.46
Ice cream, vanilla (1 cup)	540	0	170	18	138	0.92
Ice cream, vanilla, rich (1/2 cup)	476	1	87	8	70	0.3
Ice cream, vanilla, rich (1 cup)	259	2	174	16	140	0.6
Ice milk, vanilla (1/2 cup)	109	1	92	10	72	0.29
Ice milk, vanilla (1 cup)	218	2	184	20	144	0.58
Ice milk, vanilla, soft-serve (1/2 cup)	91	1	138	12	107	0.47
Ice milk, vanilla, soft-serve (1 cup)	182	2	276	24	214	0.94
Italian ice (1/2 cup)	194	1	1	0	0	0.04
Italian ice (1 cup)	388	2	2	0	0	0.08
Yogurt, chocolate, soft-serve (1/2 cup)	115	0	106	19	100	0.35
Yogurt, chocolate, soft-serve (1 cup)	230	0	206	38	200	0.7
Yogurt, vanilla, soft-serve (1/2 cup)	153	1	103	10	93	0.3
Yogurt, vanilla, soft-serve (1 cup)	306	2	206	20	186	0.6

Pastries

Ladyfingers (1 ladyfinger)	61	0	5	1	19	0.13

	VIT A (IU)	VIT C (mg)	CAL (mg)	MAG (mg)	PHOS (mg)	ZINC (mg)
Cream puffs, prepared from recipe, shell, with custard (1 cream puff)	969	0	86	16	142	0.78
Danish, fruit, enriched (1 pastry, 4¼″ dia.)	37	3	33	11	63	0.38
Danish, raspberry, unenriched (1 pastry, 4¼″ dia.)	142	3	33	11	63	0.38
Eclair, prepared from recipe, with custard (1 eclair, 5″ × 2″)	671	0	59	11	98	0.54

Pie Crust

	VIT A (IU)	VIT C (mg)	CAL (mg)	MAG (mg)	PHOS (mg)	ZINC (mg)
Cookie-type, prepared from recipe, chocolate wafer, chilled (⅛ of 9″ dia.)	235	0	8	11	29	0.23
Cookie-type, prepared from recipe, graham cracker (⅛ of 9″ dia.)	231	0	6	5	19	0.14
Standard-type, dry mix, prepared, baked (⅛ of 9″ dia.)	0	0	12	3	17	0.8
Standard-type, prepared from recipe (⅛ of 9″ dia.)	0	0	2	3	15	0.1

Pie Fillings

	VIT A (IU)	VIT C (mg)	CAL (mg)	MAG (mg)	PHOS (mg)	ZINC (mg)
Apple, canned (⅛ can)	10	1	3	2	5	0.03
Cherry, canned (⅛ can)	152	3	8	5	11	0.04

Pies

	VIT A (IU)	VIT C (mg)	CAL (mg)	MAG (mg)	PHOS (mg)	ZINC (mg)
Apple, commercially prepared, enriched flour (1 piece, ⅛ of 9″ dia.)	155	4	14	9	30	0.2

	VIT A (IU)	VIT C (mg)	CAL (mg)	MAG (mg)	PHOS (mg)	ZINC (mg)
Apple, prepared from recipe (1 piece, ⅛ of 9″ dia.)	90	3	11	11	43	0.29
Banana cream, prepared from mix no-bake type (1 piece, ⅙ of 8″ dia.)	502	1	90	15	205	0.41
Banana cream, prepared from recipe (1 piece, ⅛ of 9″ dia.)	376	2	108	23	133	0.69
Blueberry, prepared from recipe (1 piece, ⅛ of 9″ dia.)	62	1	10	12	44	0.29
Butterscotch, pudding-type, prepared from recipe (1 piece, ⅛ of 9″ dia.)	382	1	128	22	135	0.69
Cherry, prepared from recipe (1 piece ⅛ of 9″ dia.)	736	2	18	16	54	0.36
Chocolate cream, prepared from recipe (1 piece, ⅛ of 9″ dia.)	375	1	115	37	156	0.91
Coconut cream, prepared from mix, no-bake type (1 piece, ⅛ of 9″ dia.)	381	1	68	16	159	0.36
Coconut cream, prepared from recipe (1 piece, ⅛ of 9″ dia.)	380	1	113	21	140	0.81
Fried, cherry, 1 fried pie (5″ × 3¾″)	220	2	28	13	55	0.29
Lemon meringue, commercially prepared (1 piece, ⅙ of 8″ dia.)	198	4	63	17	119	0.55

	VIT A (IU)	VIT C (mg)	CAL (mg)	MAG (mg)	PHOS (mg)	ZINC (mg)
Lemon meringue, prepared from recipe (1 piece, ⅛ of 9″ dia.)	203	4	15	8	53	0.36
Mince, prepared from recipe (1 piece ⅛ of 9″ dia.)	36	10	36	23	69	0.36
Peach (1 piece, ⅙ of 8″ dia.)	123	1	9	7	29	0.11
Pecan, prepared from recipe (1 piece ⅛ of 9″ dia.)	410	0	39	32	115	1.24
Pumpkin, prepared from recipe (1 piece, ⅛ of 9″ dia.)	11,833	3	146	30	152	0.71
Vanilla cream, prepared from recipe (1 piece, ⅛ of 9″ dia.)	386	1	113	16	131	0.67

Puddings

	VIT A (IU)	VIT C (mg)	CAL (mg)	MAG (mg)	PHOS (mg)	ZINC (mg)
Banana, dry mix, instant, prepared with 2% milk (½ cup)	250	2	150	18	318	0.49
Banana, dry mix, instant, prepared with whole milk (½ cup)	154	1	147	18	315	0.47
Banana, dry mix, regular, prepared with 2% milk (½ cup)	252	1	154	18	118	0.5
Bread, prepared from recipe (½ cup)	304	1	144	24	137	0.66
Chocolate, dry mix, instant, prepared, with 2% milk (½ cup)	253	1	153	27	353	0.65
Chocolate, dry mix, instant, prepared with whole milk (½ cup)	157	1	150	27	351	0.62

	VIT A (IU)	VIT C (mg)	CAL (mg)	MAG (mg)	PHOS (mg)	ZINC (mg)
Chocolate, dry mix, regular, prepared with 2% milk (½ cup)	253	1	161	30	138	0.65
Chocolate, dry mix, regular, prepared with whole milk (½ cup)	156	1	158	21	132	0.64
Chocolate, prepared from recipe with 2% milk (½ cup)	291	1	155	39	149	0.79
Chocolate, prepared from recipe with whole milk (½ cup)	193	1	153	38	148	0.77
Lemon, dry mix, instant, with 2% milk (½ cup)	250	1	149	16	304	0.49
Lemon, dry mix, instant, with whole milk (½ cup)	154	1	146	16	301	0.47
Rice, dry mix, prepared with 2% milk (½ cup)	249	1	151	19	127	0.56
Rice, dry mix, prepared with whole milk (½ cup)	154	1	148	19	124	0.55
Rice, prepared from recipe (½ cup)	154	1	155	24	143	0.68
Tapioca, dry mix, prepared with 2% milk (½ cup)	251	1	150	17	117	0.49
Tapioca, dry mix, prepared with whole milk (½ cup)	154	1	147	17	116	0.48
Tapioca, prepared from recipe (½ cup)	315	1	158	20	160	0.75
Tapioca, ready-to-eat (½ cup)	0	1	95	9	89	0.31
Vanilla						
Dry mix, instant, prepared with 2% milk (½ cup)	241	1	146	17	183	0.47

	VIT A (IU)	VIT C (mg)	CAL (mg)	MAG (mg)	PHOS (mg)	ZINC (mg)
Dry mix, regular, prepared with 2% milk (½ cup)	252	1	153	18	118	0.5
Dry mix, regular, prepared with whole milk (½ cup)	154	1	150	18	115	0.49
Ready-to-eat (½ cup)	24	0	99	9	77	0.28
Toppings						
Butterscotch (2 tbsp.)	37	0	22	3	19	0.08
Caramel (2 tbsp.)	37	0	22	3	19	0.08
Chocolate syrup, prepared with milk (1 cup)	1126	2	292	32	229	0.92
Cream topping, whipped, pressurized (1 cup)	548	0	61	7	54	0.22
Dessert topping, powdered, 1.5 oz. (1 cup prepared)	289	1	72	8	67	0.22
Marshmallow cream (1 oz.)	0	0	1	1	2	0.01
Nuts in syrup (2 tbsp.)	17	1	16	26	46	0.43
Pineapple (2 tbsp.)	9	25	9	1	3	0.2
Rainbow Morsel Dessert Topping, Nestlé (1 packet)	1	0	4	11	13	0.15
Strawberry (2 tbsp.)	8	11	10	2	6	0.21
EGGS						
Raw, whole, fresh or frozen (1 large egg)	318	0	25	5	89	0.55
White, fresh or frozen (from 1 large egg)	0	0	2	4	4	0
Yolk, fresh or frozen (from 1 large egg)	323	0	23	1	81	0.52
Egg Beaters (¼ cup)	300	0	20	*	*	*

	VIT A (IU)	VIT C (mg)	CAL (mg)	MAG (mg)	PHOS (mg)	ZINC (mg)
Morningstar Farms Better'n Eggs (¼ cup)	640	0	7	0	29	0.51
Vegetarian, frozen (2 oz.)	311	0	2	4	4	0
Second Nature Eggs, yellow carton (¼ cup)	600	0	20	*	*	*
Second Nature Eggs, green carton (¼ cup)	500	0	40	*	*	*

FAST FOODS

Beverages

Chocolate, hot (6 oz.)	4	1	96	25	89	0.46
Float (10 oz.)	*	*	200	*	*	*
Juice, orange (6 oz.)	146	73	17	19	30	0.09
Juice, tomato (6 oz.)	1012	33	16	20	34	0.26
Malt (10 oz.)	270	4	400	*	*	*
Shakes						
Chocolate (10 oz.)	263	1	319	47	288	1.15
Strawberry (10 oz.)	340	2	320	36	283	1
Vanilla (10 oz.)	368	2	344	35	289	1.01

Breakfast

Biscuits						
Egg (1 biscuit)	649	0	154	20	185	1.1
Egg and bacon (1 biscuit)	191	3	189	24	239	1.64
Egg, cheese, and bacon (1 biscuit)	648	2	164	20	459	1.54
Ham (1 biscuit)	133	0	161	23	554	1.65
Sausage (1 biscuit)	56	0	128	20	446	1.55
Burrito (1 burrito)	1000	0	350	*	*	*
Croissant						
Egg and cheese (1 croissant)	1001	0	244	22	348	1.75

	VIT A (IU)	VIT C (mg)	CAL (mg)	MAG (mg)	PHOS (mg)	ZINC (mg)
Egg, cheese, and bacon (1 croissant)	472	2	151	23	276	1.9
Egg, cheese, and sausage (1 croissant)	422	0	144	25	290	2.15
Danish						
Cheese (1 pastry)	155	3	70	16	80	0.63
Fruit (1 pastry)	86	2	22	14	69	0.48
Egg, scrambled (2 eggs)	836	3	54	13	228	1.56
English muffin						
Butter (1 muffin)	136	1	103	13	85	0.42
Egg, cheese, and Canadian bacon (1 muffin)	594	1	207	34	320	1.81
Egg, cheese, and sausage (1 muffin)	380	1	168	24	186	1.68
French toast sticks (5 pieces)	45	0	78	27	123	0.93
Pancakes with butter and syrup (2 cakes)	281	4	128	49	476	1.02

Desserts

	VIT A (IU)	VIT C (mg)	CAL (mg)	MAG (mg)	PHOS (mg)	ZINC (mg)
Apple pie, baked (1 slice)	500	1	20	6	*	*
Banana split (1 serving)	0	18	300	*	*	*
Brownie (2″ square)	11	3	25	16	88	0.55
Cookie						
Animal crackers (1 box)	27	1	11	11	64	0.3
Chocolate chip (1 box)	52	1	20	17	52	0.34
Fried pie, fruit, apple, cherry, or lemon (1 fried pie)	149	1	13	8	37	0.17
Ice cream cone, regular (1 cone)	135	3	150	21	*	*

	VIT A (IU)	VIT C (mg)	CAL (mg)	MAG (mg)	PHOS (mg)	ZINC (mg)
Ice milk, vanilla, soft-serve, with cone (1 cone)	211	1	154	16	139	0.57
Sundae						
Caramel (1 sundae)	264	3	189	28	217	0.82
Hot fudge (1 sundae)	221	2	207	33	228	0.95
Strawberry (1 sundae)	222	2	161	25	155	0.66

Entrées

Chicken						
Breaded and fried, boneless pieces, plain (6 pieces)	102	0	16	20	204	1.06
Breaded and fried, boneless pieces with barbecue sauce (6 pieces)	342	1	21	25	215	1.12
Breaded and fried, light meat breast or wing (2 pieces)	192	0	60	38	306	1.55
Chili con carne (1 cup)	1662	2	68	46	197	3.57
Clams, breaded and fried (¾ cup)	122	0	21	31	238	1.63
Crab, soft-shell, fried (1 crab)	15	1	55	25	131	1.06
Oysters, battered or breaded and fried (6 pieces)	363	4	28	24	196	15.6
Scallops, breaded and fried (6 pieces)	138	0	19	32	292	1.08
Shrimp, breaded and fried (6–8 pieces)	120	0	84	39	344	1.21
Burrito						
Beans and cheese (1 piece)	1250	2	214	80	180	1.64
Beans and meat (2 pieces)	635	2	106	84	141	3.84

	VIT A (IU)	VIT C (mg)	CAL (mg)	MAG (mg)	PHOS (mg)	ZINC (mg)
Beans, cheese, and chili peppers (2 pieces)	1596	7	289	97	286	6.08
Beans, cheese, and beans (2 pieces)	780	5	130	51	140	2.36
Chimichanga, with beef, cheese, and red chili peppers (1 chimichanga)	702	2	218	41	148	4.63
Enchilada, with cheese (1 enchilada)	1161	1	324	51	134	2.51
Enchirito, with cheese, beef, and cheese (1 enchilada or enchirito)	1015	5	218	71	224	1.74
Taco (1 large)	1315	3	339	108	313	6.05
Tostada, with beans and cheese (1 piece)	622	1	210	59	117	1.9

Pizza

Beef (1 slice)	450	*	115	*	*	*
Cheese (1 slice)	382	1	117	16	113	0.81
Cheese, meat, and vegetables (1 slice)	524	2	101	18	131	1.12
Italian sausage (1 slice)	450	*	110	*	*	*
Pepperoni (1 slice)	282	2	65	9	75	0.52
Veggie (1 slice)	500	0	110	*	*	*

Salads

Coleslaw (¾ cup)	338	8	34	9	36	0.2
Taco (1½ cups)	588	4	192	52	143	2.69
Taco, with chili con carne (1½ cups)	1574	3	245	52	154	3.29
Vegetable salad Tossed, without dressing (1½ cups)	2352	48	27	23	81	0.44

	VIT A (IU)	VIT C (mg)	CAL (mg)	MAG (mg)	PHOS (mg)	ZINC (mg)
Tossed, without dressing, with cheese and egg (1½ cups)	822	10	100	24	132	1
Tossed, without dressing, with chicken (1½ cups)	935	17	37	33	170	0.89
Tossed, without dressing, with pasta and seafood (1½ cups)	6247	38	71	50	204	1.67
Tossed, without dressing, with shrimp (1½ cups)	791	9	59	38	161	1.27
Tossed, without dressing, with turkey, ham, and cheese (1½ cups)	1053	16	235	49	401	3.13

Sandwiches

Cheeseburger						
Patty, double, large, with condiments (1 sandwich)	462	2	111	20	176	2.09
Patty, double, large, with condiments and vegetables (1 sandwich)	348	1	240	52	395	6.68
Patty, single, regular, with condiments and vegetables (1 sandwich)	431	2	182	26	216	2.62
Chicken, broiled (1 sandwich)	150	6	75	30	*	*
Chicken fillet sandwich, plain (1 sandwich)	100	9	60	35	233	1.88
Chicken fillet, with cheese (1 sandwich)	620	3	258	43	406	2.9

	VIT A (IU)	VIT C (mg)	CAL (mg)	MAG (mg)	PHOS (mg)	ZINC (mg)
Egg and cheese (1 sandwich)	669	2	225	22	302	1.65
Fish, with tartar sauce (1 sandwich)	109	3	84	33	212	1
Fish, with tartar sauce and cheese (1 sandwich)	432	3	185	37	311	1.17
Ham and cheese (1 sandwich)	320	3	130	16	152	1.37
Hot dog, plain (1 sandwich)	0	0	24	13	97	1.98
Hot dog, with corn flour coating, corn dog (1 sandwich)	207	0	102	18	166	1.31
Roast beef, plain (1 sandwich)	210	2	54	31	239	3.39
Submarine						
Cold cuts (1 sandwich)	424	12	189	68	287	2.58
Roast beef (1 sandwich)	413	6	41	67	192	4.39
Tuna salad (1 sandwich)	187	4	74	79	335	1.87

Side dishes

	VIT A (IU)	VIT C (mg)	CAL (mg)	MAG (mg)	PHOS (mg)	ZINC (mg)
Corn, on the cob with butter (1 ear)	391	7	4	41	108	0.91
Hush puppies (5 pieces)	94	0	69	16	190	0.43
Nachos						
Cheese (6–8 nachos)	559	1	272	55	276	1.79
Cheese and jalapeño peppers (6–8 nachos)	4062	1	620	108	394	2.9
Cheese, beans, ground beef, and peppers (6–8 nachos)	3401	5	385	97	388	3.65

	VIT A (IU)	VIT C (mg)	CAL (mg)	MAG (mg)	PHOS (mg)	ZINC (mg)
Cinnamon and sugar (6–8 nachos)	108	8	85	20	33	0.59
Onion rings, breaded and fried (8–9 rings)	8	1	73	16	86	0.35
Potato						
Baked and topped with cheese, sauce (1 piece)	835	26	311	65	320	1.89
Baked and topped with cheese, sauce, and bacon (1 piece)	628	29	308	69	347	2.15
Baked and topped with cheese, sauce, and broccoli (1 piece)	1695	49	336	78	346	2.03
Baked and topped with cheese, sauce, and chili (1 piece)	766	32	411	111	498	3.79
Baked and topped with sour cream and chives (1 piece)	1347	34	106	70	184	0.91
French fried in vegetable oil (1 large potato)	33	6	18	38	153	0.6
Mashed (1/3 cup)	33	0	17	14	44	0.26

FATS

Butter

	VIT A (IU)	VIT C (mg)	CAL (mg)	MAG (mg)	PHOS (mg)	ZINC (mg)
Blend, corn oil and butter (1 tbsp.)	507	0	4	0	3	0
Regular (1 tbsp.)	434	0	3	0	3	0.01
Whipped (1 tbsp.)	288	0	2	0	2	0.01

Margarine/ Spreads	VIT A (IU)	VIT C (mg)	CAL (mg)	MAG (mg)	PHOS (mg)	ZINC (mg)
Hard, soybean, regular, hydrogenated (1 tsp.)	168	0	1	0	1	0
Imitation, soybean, hydrogenated (1 tsp.)	171	0	1	0	1	0
Liquid, soybean and cottonseed, hydrogenated and regular (1 tsp.)	168	0	3	0	2	0
Soft, corn, hydrogenated and regular (1 tsp.)	168	0	1	0	1	0
Soft, soybean, hydrogenated and regular (1 tsp.)	168	0	1	0	1	0
Soft spread, Smart Balance, GFA Brands (1 tbsp.)	500	*	*	*	*	*
Soybean, soft, hydrogenated and regular (1 tsp.)	168	0	1	0	1	0
Spread, tub, soybean and cottonseed oil, hydrogenated (1 tsp.)	171	0	1	0	1	0
Mayonnaise						
Imitation, milk cream (1 tbsp.)	2	0	11	1	9	0.04
Imitation, soybean (1 tbsp.)	0	0	0	0	0	0.02
Imitation, soybean, without cholesterol (1 tbsp.)	0	0	0	0	0	0.02
Regular (1 tbsp.)	32	0	2	0	4	0.03
Soybean oil (1 tbsp.)	39	0	3	0	4	0.02
Oil						
Canola (1 tbsp.)	0	0	0	0	0	0
Corn, salad or cooking (1 tbsp.)	0	0	0	0	0	0

	VIT A (IU)	VIT C (mg)	CAL (mg)	MAG (mg)	PHOS (mg)	ZINC (mg)
Cottonseed, salad or cooking (1 tbsp.)	0	0	0	0	0	0
Olive, salad or cooking (1 tbsp.)	0	0	0	0	0	0.01
Peanut, salad or cooking (1 tbsp.)	0	0	0	0	0	0
Safflower, salad or cooking (1 tbsp.)	0	0	0	0	0	0
Sesame, salad or cooking (1 tbsp.)	0	0	0	0	0	0
Soybean, salad or cooking, hydrogenated (1 tbsp.)	0	0	0	0	0	0
Sunflower (1 tbsp.)	0	0	0	0	0	0
Tomatoseed (1 tbsp.)	0	0	0	0	0	0
Wheat germ (1 tbsp.)	0	0	0	0	0	0

FRUIT

	VIT A (IU)	VIT C (mg)	CAL (mg)	MAG (mg)	PHOS (mg)	ZINC (mg)
Acerola, West Indian cherry, raw (1 cup)	752	1655	12	18	11	0.09
Apples						
Dried, uncooked (1 ring)	0	0	1	1	2	0.01
Frozen, unsweetened (1 cup)	59	0	7	5	14	0.09
Raw, with skin (1 medium)	73	8	10	7	10	0.06
Apricots						
Dried, stewed, without sugar (½ cup)	2954	2	20	22	52	0.33
Dried, stewed, without sugar (1 cup)	5908	4	40	43	103	0.65
Frozen, sweeten (1 cup)	4066	22	24	22	46	0.24
Raw (1 apricot)	914	4	5	3	7	0.09
Avocados, raw (1 cup)	894	12	16	57	60	0.61
Bananas, raw (½ medium)	48	6	4	17	12	0.099

	VIT A (IU)	VIT C (mg)	CAL (mg)	MAG (mg)	PHOS (mg)	ZINC (mg)
Bananas, raw (1 medium)	96	11	7	34	24	0.19
Blackberries						
Frozen, unsweetened (½ cup)	86	2.5	22	17	23	0.29
Frozen, unsweetened (1 cup)	172	5	44	33	45	0.38
Raw (½ cup)	129	15	23	15	15	0.19
Raw (1 cup)	238	30	46	29	30	0.39
Blueberries						
Frozen, sweetened (1 cup)	101	2	14	5	16	0.14
Frozen, unsweetened (½ cup)	63	2	6	4	8.5	0.06
Frozen, unsweetened (1 cup)	126	4	12	8	17	0.11
Raw (½ cup)	73	9	5	4	8	0.08
Raw (1 cup)	145	19	9	7	15	0.16
Breadfruit, raw (¼ small fruit)	38	28	16	24	29	0.12
Cantaloupe, raw (1 cup cubes)	5158	68	18	18	27	0.26
Casaba, raw (1 cup cubes)	51	27	9	14	12	0.27
Cherimoya, raw, without skin and seeds (1 fruit)	55	49	126	218	*	*
Cherries						
Sour, red, raw without pits (1 cup)	1989	16	25	14	23	0.16
Sweet, raw, without pits (1 cup)	310	10	22	16	28	0.09
Sweet, frozen, thawed (1 cup)	490	3	31	26	41	0.1
Coconut meat, raw (1 cup shredded)	0	3	11	26	90	0.88
Crabapples, raw (1 cup slices)	44	9	20	8	17	*
Currants, European black, raw (1 cup)	258	203	62	27	66	0.3

	VIT A (IU)	VIT C (mg)	CAL (mg)	MAG (mg)	PHOS (mg)	ZINC (mg)
Currants, red and white, raw (1 cup)	134	46	37	15	49	0.26
Dates, domestic, natural and dry (1 cup, pitted)	89	0	57	62	71	0.52
Figs, dried, stewed (1 cup)	412	11	158	65	75	0.54
Figs, raw (1 medium)	71	1	18	9	7	0.08
Fruit, mixed, peach, cherry (sweet and sour), raspberry, grape, and boysenberry, frozen, sweetened (1 cup thawed)	805	188	18	15	30	0.13
Gooseberries, raw (1 cup)	435	42	38	15	41	0.18
Grapefruit, raw, pink, red, and white, all areas (½ large)	206	57	20	13	13	0.12
Grapes, American type, slip skin, raw (1 cup)	92	4	13	5	9	0.04
Honeydew, raw (1 cup, diced)	68	42	10	12	17	0.12
Jackfruit, raw (100 g)	297	6.7	34	37	36	0.42
Kiwi fruit, Chinese gooseberries, raw (1 large fruit without skin)	160	90	24	27	36	0.16
Mangos, raw (1 cup, sliced)	6425	46	17	15	18	0.07
Mulberries, raw (1 cup)	35	51	55	25	53	0.17
Nectarines, raw (1 cup, sliced)	1016	7	7	11	22	0.12
Oranges, raw (1 fruit)	269	70	52	13	18	0.09
Papayas, raw (1 medium)	863	188	73	30	15	0.21
Passion fruit, purple, raw (1 fruit, sliced)	126	5	2	5	12	0.02

	VIT A (IU)	VIT C (mg)	CAL (mg)	MAG (mg)	PHOS (mg)	ZINC (mg)
Peaches						
Dried, stewed, without sugar (1 cup)	508	10	23	34	98	0.46
Raw (1 medium)	524	7	5	7	12	0.14
Frozen, sliced, sweetened (1 cup, thawed)	710	236	8	13	28	0.13
Pears, dried, stewed, without added sugar (1 cup, halves)	107	10	41	41	71	0.49
Pears, raw (1 medium fruit)	33	7	18	10	18	0.2
Plantains, cooked (1 cup, sliced)	1400	17	3	49	43	0.2
Plantains, raw (1 cup, sliced)	1668	27	4	55	50	0.2
Plums, raw (1 fruit)	213	6	3	5	7	0.07
Pomegranates, raw (1 fruit)	0	9	5	5	12	0.19
Prunes, dehydrated, uncooked (1 cup)	2326	0	95	85	148	0.99
Prunes, dried, stewed, without sugar (1 cup, pitted)	759	7	57	50	87	0.6
Raisins, golden seedless (1 cup)	64	5	77	51	167	0.46
Raisins, seedless (1 cup, not packed)	12	5	71	48	141	0.39
Raspberries, frozen, red, sweetened (1 cup, unthawed)	150	41	38	33	43	0.45
Raspberries, raw (1 cup)	160	31	27	22	15	0.57
Rhubarb, frozen, cooked, with sugar (1 cup)	166	8	348	29	19	0.19
Rhubarb, raw (1 cup, diced)	122	10	105	15	17	0.12

	VIT A (IU)	VIT C (mg)	CAL (mg)	MAG (mg)	PHOS (mg)	ZINC (mg)
Strawberries, frozen, sweetened, whole (1 cup, thawed)	69	101	28	15	31	0.13
Strawberries, frozen, unsweetened (1 cup, thawed)	100	91	35	24	29	0.29
Strawberries, raw (1 cup, whole)	39	82	20	14	27	0.19
Tamarindo, tart date-apricot flavored fruit (3 oz.)	0	4	60	*	*	*
Tangerines, raw (1 medium fruit)	773	26	12	10	8	0.2
Watermelon, raw (1 cup, diced)	556	15	12	17	14	0.11

Canned Fruit

	VIT A (IU)	VIT C (mg)	CAL (mg)	MAG (mg)	PHOS (mg)	ZINC (mg)
Apples, sweetened, sliced, drained (1 cup)	104	1	8	4	10	0.06
Applesauce, sweetened (1 cup)	28	4	10	8	18	0.1
Apricots, juice pack, with skin (1 cup, halves)	4126	12	29	24	49	0.27
Apricots, water pack, with skin (1 cup)	3142	8	19	17	32	0.27
Blackberries, heavy syrup (1 cup)	561	7	54	44	35	0.46
Blueberries, heavy syrup (1 cup)	164	3	13	10	26	0.18
Cherries, sour, red, light syrup pack (1 cup)	1830	5	25	15	25	0.18
Cherries, sour, red, water pack, solids and liquids (1 cup)	1840	5	27	15	24	0.17
Cherries, sweet, water pack (1 cup)	397	5	27	22	37	0.2

	VIT A (IU)	VIT C (mg)	CAL (mg)	MAG (mg)	PHOS (mg)	ZINC (mg)
Figs, light syrup pack (1 cup)	93	3	68	25	25	0.28
Fruit cocktail, peach, pineapple, pear, grape, and cherry, juice packed (1 cup)	723	6	19	17	33	0.21
Fruit salad, peach, pear, apricot, pineapple, and cherry, juice pack (1 cup)	1494	8	27	20	35	0.35
Gooseberries, light syrup pack (1 cup)	348	25	40	15	18	0.28
Grapefruit, sections, juice pack (1 cup)	0	84	37	27	30	0.2
Orange-grapefruit juice, unsweetened (1 cup)	294	72	20	25	35	0.17
Papaya nectar (1 cup)	278	8	25	8	0	0.37
Peaches, juice pack (1 cup)	945	9	15	17	42	0.27
Pears, juice pack (1 cup)	5	1	7	5	9	0.07
Pineapple, juice pack (1 cup)	95	24	35	35	15	0.25
Plums, purple, juice pack (1 cup, pitted)	2543	7	25	20	38	0.28
Raspberries, red, heavy syrup (1 cup)	85	22	28	31	23	0.41
Strawberries, heavy syrup pack (1 cup)	66	81	33	20	31	0.23
Tangerines (or mandarin oranges), juice pack (1 cup)	2122	85	27	27	25	1.27

Fruit Juices

	VIT A (IU)	VIT C (mg)	CAL (mg)	MAG (mg)	PHOS (mg)	ZINC (mg)
Apple cider, canned (1 cup)	*	6000	*	*	*	*
Apple juice Canned, unsweetened, with added ascorbic acid (1 cup)	3	103	17	7	17	0.07

	VIT A (IU)	VIT C (mg)	CAL (mg)	MAG (mg)	PHOS (mg)	ZINC (mg)
Canned, unsweetened (1 cup)	3	2	17	7	17	0.07
Frozen concentrate (1 cup)	0	60	14	12	17	0.1
Apricot nectar, canned (1 cup)	3304	1	17	13	23	0.23
Carrot juice, canned (1 cup)	60,772	20	57	33	99	0.43
Carrot, Apple, and Tropical Fruit Blend, V-8, 25% juice (1 cup)	5000	60	*	*	*	*
Citrus fruit juice drink, frozen concentrate, prepared (1 cup)	104	67	22	15	25	0.12
Clam and tomato juice, canned (1 can, 5.5 oz.)	357	7	20	37	130	1.79
Cranberry-apple juice drink, bottled (1 cup)	7	78	17	5	7	0.1
Cranberry-apricot juice drink, bottled (1 cup)	1134	0	22	7	12	0.1
Cranberry-grape juice drink, bottled (1 cup)	12	78	20	7	10	0.1
Cranberry juice cocktail, bottled (1 cup)	10	90	8	5	5	0.18
Cranberry juice cocktail, bottled, low calorie, with calcium (1 cup)	10	76	21	5	2	0.05
Cranberry juice cocktail, frozen, concentrate, prepared (1 cup)	25	25	13	5	3	0.1
Grape juice, canned or bottled, unsweetened, without added vitamin C (1 cup)	20	0	23	25	28	0.13
Grape juice, frozen concentrate, sweetened (1 cup)	20	60	10	10	10	0.1
Grape juice drink, canned (1 cup)	5	40	8	10	10	0.08

	VIT A (IU)	VIT C (mg)	CAL (mg)	MAG (mg)	PHOS (mg)	ZINC (mg)
Grapefruit juice, canned, sweetened (1 cup)	0	67	20	25	28	0.15
Grapefruit juice, frozen concentrate, unsweetened, undiluted (1 can, 6 oz.)	64	248	56	79	101	0.37
Grapefruit juice, pink, raw (1 cup)	1087	94	22	30	37	0.12
Grapefruit juice, white, raw (1 cup)	25	94	22	30	37	0.12
Lemonade, powder, prepared with water (1 cup)	0	8	71	3	34	0.11
Lemon juice, canned or bottled (1 oz.)	5	8	3	2	3	0.02
Lemon juice, raw (juice of 1 lemon)	9	22	3	3	3	0.02
Lime juice, canned or bottled, unsweetened (1 oz.)	5	2	4	2	3	0.02
Lime juice, raw (1 oz.)	3	9	3	2	2	0.02
Orange-apricot juice drink, canned (1 cup)	1450	50	13	10	20	0.13
Orange-grapefruit juice, canned, unsweetened (1 cup)	294	72	20	25	35	0.17
Orange juice						
Canned, unsweetened (1 cup)	435	86	20	26	35	0.17
From concentrate, Season's Best, Tropicana (1 cup)	0	60	300	*	*	*
Frozen concentrate, unsweetened, diluted with water (1 cup)	194	97	22	25	40	0.13
Raw (1 cup)	496	124	27	27	42	0.12

	VIT A (IU)	VIT C (mg)	CAL (mg)	MAG (mg)	PHOS (mg)	ZINC (mg)
Squeezed, Not From Concentrate Plus Calcium, Florida's Natural Brand, Citrus World (1 cup)	*	108	350	31	41	.01
Squeezed, Not from Concentrate Calcium Enriched, Tropicana (1 cup)	*	108	350	*	*	*
Papaya nectar, canned (1 cup)	278	8	25	8	0	0.38
Passion fruit juice, raw (1 cup)	1771	74	10	42	32	0.12
Passion fruit juice, yellow, raw (1 cup)	5953	45	10	42	62	0.15
Peach nectar, canned, with added ascorbic acid (1 cup)	642	67	13	10	15	0.2
Pear nectar, canned, with added ascorbic acid (1 cup)	3	68	13	8	8	0.18
Pineapple juice, canned, with added ascorbic acid, unsweetened (1 cup)	13	60	43	33	20	0.28
Pineapple juice, frozen concentrate, unsweetened, diluted with water (1 cup)	25	30	28	23	20	0.28
Pineapple-grapefruit juice drink, canned (1 cup)	88	115	18	15	15	0.15
Pineapple-orange juice drink, canned (1 cup)	1328	56	13	15	10	0.15
Prune juice, canned (1 cup)	8	11	31	36	64	0.54
Tangerine juice, canned, sweetened (1 cup)	1046	55	45	20	35	0.08

	VIT A (IU)	VIT C (mg)	CAL (mg)	MAG (mg)	PHOS (mg)	ZINC (mg)
Tangerine juice, frozen concentrate, sweetened, diluted with water (1 cup)	1381	59	19	19	19	0.07
Tangerine juice, frozen concentrate, sweetened, undiluted (6 oz.)	4310	182	58	60	64	0.19
Tangerine juice, raw (1 cup)	1037	77	45	20	35	0.07
Tomato juice, canned, with salt added (1 cup)	1351	45	22	27	46	0.34
Tomato juice, canned, without salt added (1 cup)	1351	45	22	27	46	0.34
Vegetable juice cocktail, canned (1 cup)	2831	67	27	27	41	0.48

GRAVIES, SAUCES, AND DIPS

Gravies

	VIT A (IU)	VIT C (mg)	CAL (mg)	MAG (mg)	PHOS (mg)	ZINC (mg)
Au jus, canned (1 cup)	0	2	10	5	72	2.38
Beef, canned (1 cup)	0	0	14	5	70	2.33
Chicken, canned (1 cup)	878	0	48	5	69	1.9
Mushroom, canned (1 cup)	0	0	17	5	36	1.67
Turkey gravy mix, canned (1 cup)	0	0	10	5	70	2
Turkey Gravy Mix, Nestlé, Trio, dry (1 serving)	0	0	10	5	29	0.01

Sauces

	VIT A (IU)	VIT C (mg)	CAL (mg)	MAG (mg)	PHOS (mg)	ZINC (mg)
Alfredo, dry, Nestlé, Trio (100 g)	567	0	467	32	415	1.49
Barbecue (1 packet)	81	1	2	2	2	0.02

	VIT A (IU)	VIT C (mg)	CAL (mg)	MAG (mg)	PHOS (mg)	ZINC (mg)
Béarnaise, dehydrated, dry (1 cup)	1	0	27	5	24	0.12
Cheese						
Cheddar, basic, Nestlé, Chef-Mate ready-to-serve (¼ cup)	39	1	46	4	51	0.34
Jalapeño, Nestlé, Que Bueno (¼ cup)	71	1	54	4	52	0.34
Mix, dry, Nestlé, Trio (2 tbsp.)	21	0	22	4	34	0.13
Sharp cheddar, Nestlé, Chef-Mate ready-to-serve (1 cup)	1210	0	544	25	421	2.6
Chili, hot dog sauce, ready-to-serve Nestlé, Chef-Mate (¼ cup)	423	0	20	13	40	0.55
Cranberry sauce, canned, sweetened (1 slice)	11	1	2	2	3	0.03
Creole, ready-to-serve, Nestlé, Chef-Mate (¼ cup)	234	0	35	9	17	0.1
Curry, dehydrated, dry (1 cup)	29	1	50	12	42	0.26
Enchilada, ready-to-serve, Nestlé, Que Bueno (2 tbsp.)	123	2	7	5	11	0.06
Guava, cooked (1 cup)	674	348	17	17	26	0.41
Hollandaise, with butterfat, dehydrated, dry (1 packet)	573	0	97	6	99	0.54
Lemon, ready-to-serve, Nestlé, Chef-Mate (2 tbsp.)	0	3	1	1	1	0.01

	VIT A (IU)	VIT C (mg)	CAL (mg)	MAG (mg)	PHOS (mg)	ZINC (mg)
Marinara, ready-to-serve (½ cup)	469	10	28	21	40	0.21
Pesto (¼ package)	300	*	20	*	*	*
Plum, ready-to-serve (1 tbsp.)	8	0	2	2	4	0.04
Sour cream, dehydrated, dry (1 tbsp.)	85	0	128	7	42	0.64
Spaghetti sauce, ready-to-serve, Nestlé, Contadine (½ cup)	500	11	31	28	46	0.26
Stir fry sauce, Nestlé, Chef-Mate, all purpose (1 tbsp.)	4	1	2	2	5	0.02
Stroganoff, dehydrated, dry (1 cup)	268	0	371	23	152	1.33
Sweet and sour, dehydrated, dry (1 cup)	0	0	41	9	45	0.09
Szechuan, ready-to-serve, Nestlé Chef-Mate (2 tbsp.)	197	1	4	3	12	0.04
Teriyaki, ready-to-serve, Nestlé, Chef-Mate (1 tbsp.)	0	0	1	1	3	0.02
Tomato, canned (1 cup)	2399	32	34	47	78	0.61
White, homemade sauce						
Medium (½ cup)	691	1	148	18	123	0.51
Thick (½ cup)	841	1	139	18	120	0.5
Thin (½ cup)	504	1	158	19	126	0.53

Dips

	VIT A (IU)	VIT C (mg)	CAL (mg)	MAG (mg)	PHOS (mg)	ZINC (mg)
Cheese, prepared (1 cup)	1473	2	756	46	557	0.06
Cheese, fondue (1 cup)	890	0	1023	50	658	4.21
Con Queso, Nestlé, Que Bueno (¼ cup)	172	0	118	4	52	0.33

	VIT A (IU)	VIT C (mg)	CAL (mg)	MAG (mg)	PHOS (mg)	ZINC (mg)
Garden vegetable, prepared (1 tbsp.)	200	2	40	*	*	*
Nacho, Nestlé, Que Bueno (¼ cup)	481	0	181	6	105	0.65
Ranch, fat-free, prepared with fat-free sour cream (1/16 packet)	200	0	60	*	*	*
Ranch, prepared (1/16 packet)	200	0	20	*	*	*
Picante, ready-to-serve, Nestlé, Que Bueno (2 tbsp.)	83	1	13	5	8	0.05
Salsa, creamy, fat-free, prepared (2 tbsp.)	*	*	60	*	*	*
Salsa, ready-to-serve (½ cup)	862	26	60	16	30	0.38

MEATS

Beef

	VIT A (IU)	VIT C (mg)	CAL (mg)	MAG (mg)	PHOS (mg)	ZINC (mg)
Brisket, whole, lean and fat, all grades, braised (3 oz.)	0	0	7	15	159	4.34
Chuck, arm pot roast, lean and fat, choice, braised (3 oz.)	0	0	9	16	184	5.7
Chuck, blade roast, lean and fat, choice, braised (3 oz.)	0	0	15	26	223	9.23
Corn beef, cured, canned (100 g)	0	0	12	14	106	3.87
Flank, lean only, choice, braised (3 oz.)	0	0	5	20	227	5.14
Ground, lean, pan-fried, medium (3 oz.)	0	0	6	18	136	4.61
Liver, braised (3 oz.)	30,327	20	6	17	343	5.16
Liver, pan-fried (3 oz.)	30,589	20	9	20	392	4.63

	VIT A (IU)	VIT C (mg)	CAL (mg)	MAG (mg)	PHOS (mg)	ZINC (mg)
Porterhouse short loin, steak, lean, choice, broiled (3 oz.)	0	0	6	23	179	4.5
Porterhouse steak, short loin, lean and fat, choice, broiled (3 oz.)	0	0	7	19	152	3.7
Rib eye, small end (ribs 10–12), lean and fat, choice, broiled (3 oz.)	3	0	11	20	156	5.08
Round, bottom round, lean and fat, choice, braised (3 oz.)	0	0	5	19	208	4.17
Round, tip round, lean and fat, choice, roasted (3 oz.)	0	0	5	20	189	5.43
T-bone steak, short loin, all grades, broiled (3 oz.)	0	0	7	20	159	3.83
T-bone steak, short loin, choice, broiled (3 oz.)	0	0	7	20	156	3.78
T-bone steak, short loin, lean and fat, choice, broiled (3 oz.)	0	0	6	21	168	4.11
T-bone steak, short loin, lean, choice, broiled (3 oz.)	0	0	5	24	183	4.51
Tenderloin, lean and fat, choice, broiled (3 oz.)	0	0	7	22	178	4.11
Top sirloin, lean and fat, choice, broiled (3 oz.)	0	0	9	24	187	4.93

Game Meat

	VIT A (IU)	VIT C (mg)	CAL (mg)	MAG (mg)	PHOS (mg)	ZINC (mg)
Beefalo, composite of cuts, roasted (3 oz.)	0	8	20	213	390	5.44
Bison, roasted (3 oz.)	0	0	7	22	178	3.13
Buffalo, roasted (3 oz.)	0	0	13	28	187	2.16
Rabbit, composite of cuts, roasted (3 oz.)	0	0	16	18	224	1.93

Lamb	VIT A (IU)	VIT C (mg)	CAL (mg)	MAG (mg)	PHOS (mg)	ZINC (mg)
Ground, broiled (3 oz.)	0	0	19	20	171	3.97
Leg, domestic, sirloin half, lean and fat, choice, roasted (3 oz.)	0	0	9	19	156	3.51
Loin, domestic, lean only, choice, broiled (3 oz.)	0	0	16	24	192	3.51
Liver, braised (3 oz.)	21,203	3	7	19	357	6.71
Luncheon Meats						
Beef, thin sliced (5 slices)	0	0	2	4	35	0.84
Bologna, beef (1 slice)	0	0	3	3	20	0.5
Bologna, turkey (2 slices)	0	0	48	8	74	0.99
Ham, extra lean, 5% fat (1 slice)	0	0	2	5	62	0.55
Ham, regular, 11% fat (1 slice)	0	0	2	5	70	0.61
Pastrami, beef, cured (100 g)	0	0	9	18	150	4.26
Pastrami, turkey (2 slices)	0	0	5	8	113	1.23
Salami						
Beef, cooked (1 slice)	0	0	2	3	26	0.5
Beef, beer, beerwurst (1 slice)	0	0	2	3	22	0.56
Pork, beer, beerwurst (1 slice)	0	0	2	3	24	0.4
Pork, beef, dry or hard (1 slice)	0	0	1	2	14	0.32
Turkey, cooked (2 slices)	0	0	11	9	60	1.03
Pork						
Bacon, Canadian-style, grilled (2 slices)	0	0	5	10	138	0.79

	VIT A (IU)	VIT C (mg)	CAL (mg)	MAG (mg)	PHOS (mg)	ZINC (mg)
Bacon, cured, cooked, broiled, pan-fried, or roasted (3 med. slices)	0	0	2	5	64	0.62
Ham						
Cured, boneless, extra lean, 5% fat (3 oz.)	0	0	7	12	167	2.45
Cured, extra lean, 4% fat, canned, roasted (3 oz.)	0	0	5	18	178	1.9
Patties, grilled (1 patty)	0	0	5	6	60	1.13
Steak, cured, boneless, extra lean (1 slice)	0	18	2	11	147	1.15

Sausage

	VIT A (IU)	VIT C (mg)	CAL (mg)	MAG (mg)	PHOS (mg)	ZINC (mg)
Bockwurst, pork, veal, uncooked (1 link)	15	0	10	12	95	1.01
Chorizo, pork and beef (1 link)	0	0	5	11	90	2.05
Frankfurter, beef (1 frankfurter)	0	0	9	1	39	0.98
Frankfurter, beef and pork (1 frankfurter)	0	0	5	5	39	0.83
Frankfurter, turkey (1 frankfurter)	0	0	48	6	60	1.4
Keilbasa, kolbassy, pork, beef, nonfat dry milk added (1 slice)	0	0	11	4	39	0.53
Link, smoked, pork (1 link)	0	1	20	13	110	1.92
Link, smoked, pork and beef, nonfat dry milk added (1 link)	0	0	28	11	93	1.33

Veal

	VIT A (IU)	VIT C (mg)	CAL (mg)	MAG (mg)	PHOS (mg)	ZINC (mg)
Ground, broiled (3 oz.)	0	0	15	20	185	3.29

	VIT A (IU)	VIT C (mg)	CAL (mg)	MAG (mg)	PHOS (mg)	ZINC (mg)
Leg, top round, lean and fat, braised (100 g)	0	0	8	29	249	3.96
Loin, lean and fat, braised (3 oz.)	0	0	24	20	187	3.09
Sirloin, lean only, braised (3 oz.)	0	0	16	25	220	4.04

Vegetarian, Meatless

	VIT A (IU)	VIT C (mg)	CAL (mg)	MAG (mg)	PHOS (mg)	ZINC (mg)
Bacon (1 strip)	4	0	1	1	4	0.02
Breakfast Patties, Morningstar Farms (1 patty)	0	0	18	1	106	0.37
Burgers, meatless						
Black Bean, spicy, Morningstar Farms (1 patty)	139	0	56	44	150	0.93
Crumbles, Morningstar Farms (1 cup)	0	0	79	2	174	1.64
Garden Vege Patties, Morningstar Farms (1 patty)	766	0	48	30	124	0.58
Harvest Burgers, Green Giant (⅔ cup)	0	0	100	*	*	4.5
Vegan, Morningstar Farms (1 patty)	0	0	87	16	181	0.75
Veggie Burgers, Yves (1 patty)	100	0	60	*	*	*
Deli slices, Veggie, Yves (3.5 slices)	0	0	30	*	*	*
Franks, Deli, Morningstar Farms (1 serving)	0	0	17	4	42	0.38
Sausage, meatless (1 patty)	243	0	24	14	86	0.56
Tofu Crumbles, Vegetarian Hamburgers, Marjon (2½ oz.)	0	0	60	*	*	*

	VIT A (IU)	VIT C (mg)	CAL (mg)	MAG (mg)	PHOS (mg)	ZINC (mg)
Wieners, Veggie, Yves (1 link)	0	0	20	*	*	*

MILK, CREAM, AND YOGURT

Milk

	VIT A (IU)	VIT C (mg)	CAL (mg)	MAG (mg)	PHOS (mg)	ZINC (mg)
1%, protein fortified, with added vitamin A (1 cup)	499	3	349	39	273	1.11
1%, with added nonfat solids and vitamin A (1 cup)	500	3	313	35	245	0.98
2%, protein fortified, with added vitamin A (1 cup)	500	3	352	40	276	1.11
2%, with added nonfat milk solids and vitamin A (1 cup)	500	3	313	35	245	0.98
3.3%, whole (1 cup)	307	2	291	33	228	0.93
Buttermilk, dried (1 tbsp.)	14	0	77	7	61	0.26
Buttermilk, fluid, cultured, from skim milk (1 cup)	81	2	285	27	219	1.03
CalciMilk, nonfat, A & D added (1 cup)	500	0	500	*	*	*
Chocolate beverage, hot cocoa, homemade (1 cup)	515	3	315	70	293	1.48
Chocolate dairy drink mix, with aspartame, prepared with water (1 pkg., ½ cup water, 3 ice cubes)	120	0	94	23	89	0.4
Chocolate drink, fluid, commercial, 1% (1 cup)	500	2	287	33	257	1.03
Chocolate drink, fluid, commercial, 2% (1 cup)	500	2	284	33	254	1.03

	VIT A (IU)	VIT C (mg)	CAL (mg)	MAG (mg)	PHOS (mg)	ZINC (mg)
Chocolate drink, fluid, commercial, whole (1 cup)	303	2	280	33	251	1.03
Condensed, sweetened, canned (1 cup)	1004	8	868	79	775	2.88
Dry, skim, nonfat solids, instant, with added vitamin A (⅓ cup)	545	1	283	27	227	1.01
Dry, skim, nonfat solids, regular, with added vitamin A (1 cup)	659	2	377	33	291	1.22
Dry, whole (¼ cup)	295	3	292	27	248	1.07
Dairy drink, chocolate, reduced-calorie, with aspartame, powder, prepared with water (6 oz.)	245	0	192	47	182	0.82
Evaporated, skim, canned (1 cup)	1004	3	741	69	499	2.3
Evaporated, whole, with added vitamin A (½ cup)	500	2	329	31	255	0.97
Evaporated, whole, without added vitamin A (1 cup)	612	5	657	61	510	1.94
Goat, fluid (1 cup)	451	3	326	34	270	0.73
Lactose-free (1 cup)	500	*	300	*	*	*
Lactose-reduced (1 cup)	*	*	300	*	*	*
Lactose-reduced, calcium-fortified (1 cup)	*	*	500	*	*	*
Parmalat, whole, long life (½ pint)	300	3	300	*	*	*
Rice Dream, rice beverage, Imagine Foods (1 cup)	500	0	300	*	*	*
Shake, chocolate, thick (10.6 oz.)	258	0	396	48	378	1.44
Shake, vanilla, thick (11 oz.)	357	0	457	37	361	1.22

	VIT A (IU)	VIT C (mg)	CAL (mg)	MAG (mg)	PHOS (mg)	ZINC (mg)
Skim, protein fortified, with added vitamin A (1 cup)	499	3	352	40	275	1.11
Skim, with added nonfat milk solids and vitamin A (1 cup)	500	3	316	36	255	1
Soy milk (1 cup)	78	0	10	47	120	0.56
Soy Moo, fat-free, nondairy, lactose-free (1 cup)	0	0	400	*	*	*
Whole, low-sodium (1 cup)	317	2	246	12	209	0.93
Vitamite, 2% fat, nondairy, 100% lactose-free, added calcium and milk protein (1 cup)	500	0	200	*	100	*

Cream

	VIT A (IU)	VIT C (mg)	CAL (mg)	MAG (mg)	PHOS (mg)	ZINC (mg)
Cream topping, whipped, pressurized (1 tbsp.)	27	0	3	0	3	0.01
Half and half (1 oz.)	131	0	32	3	29	0.15
Heavy, whipping, fluid (1 oz.)	438	0	19	2	19	0.07
Light, coffee or table, fluid (1 oz.)	216	0	29	3	24	0.08
Light, whipping, fluid (1 tbsp.)	169	0	10	1	9	0.04
Sour, cultured (1 tbsp.)	95	0	14	1	10	0.03
Sour dressing, nonbutterfat, cultured, filled cream-type (1 tbsp.)	1	0	14	1	11	0.04
Sour, half and half, cultured (1 tbsp.)	68	0	16	2	14	0.08
Sour, imitation, cultured (1 oz.)	0	0	1	2	13	0.34

Yogurt	VIT A (IU)	VIT C (mg)	CAL (mg)	MAG (mg)	PHOS (mg)	ZINC (mg)
Coffee, low-fat, 11 g protein per 1 cup (1 cup)	132	2	420	40	330	2.03
Fruit, low-fat, 9 g protein per 1 cup (1 cup)	120	2	339	33	266	1.64
Fruit, low-fat, 10 g protein per 1 cup (1 cup)	104	2	345	33	271	1.68
Fruit, low-fat, 11 g protein per 1 cup (1 cup)	136	2	383	37	301	1.86
Frozen, chocolate, soft-serve (½ cup)	115	0	106	19	100	0.35
Frozen, vanilla, soft-serve (½ cup)	153	1	103	10	93	0.3
Plain, fat-free (1 cup)	0	0	400	*	*	*
Plain, low-fat, 12 g protein per 1 cup (1 cup)	162	2	447	43	352	2.18
Plain, skim milk, 13 g protein per 1 cup (1 cup)	17	2	488	47	383	2.38
Plain, whole milk, 8 g protein per 1 cup (1 cup)	301	1	296	28	233	1.45

MISCELLANEOUS

Condiments

	VIT A (IU)	VIT C (mg)	CAL (mg)	MAG (mg)	PHOS (mg)	ZINC (mg)
Catsup (1 tbsp.)	152	2	3	3	6	0.04
Catsup, low-sodium (1 tbsp.)	152	2	3	3	6	0.04
Mayonnaise (1 tbsp.)	32	0	2	*	4	*
Mustard, yellow (1 tbsp.)	0	*	4	*	4	*
Pepper sauce, hot (¼ tsp.)	4	1	0	0	0	0
Pickle, cucumber, dill (1 spear)	99	1	3	3	6	0.04

	VIT A (IU)	VIT C (mg)	CAL (mg)	MAG (mg)	PHOS (mg)	ZINC (mg)
Pickle, cucumber, sweet (1 pickle)	3	0	1	1	3	0.02
Pickle relish						
Hamburger (1 tbsp.)	40	0	1	1	3	0.02
Hot dog (1 tbsp.)	25	0	1	3	6	0.03
Sweet (1 tbsp.)	23	0	1	1	2	0.02
Soy sauce (1 tbsp.)	0	0	3	6	20	0.07
Soy sauce, made from soy and wheat (shoyu), low-sodium (1 tbsp.)	0	0	3	6	20	0.07
Soy sauce, made from soy, tamari (1 tbsp.)	0	0	4	7	23	0.08
Tahini, sesame butter (1 oz.)	19	0	121	27	208	1.31
Tabasco, pepper, ready-to-serve (¼ tsp.)	20	0	0	0	0	0
Tartar sauce (1 tbsp.)	30	*	3	*	4	*
Teriyaki (1 tbsp.)	0	0	4	11	28	0.02
Vinegar, cider (1 tbsp.)	0	0	1	*	1	*

Leavening Agents

	VIT A (IU)	VIT C (mg)	CAL (mg)	MAG (mg)	PHOS (mg)	ZINC (mg)
Baking powder, double-acting, low-sodium (1 tsp.)	0	0	216	1	343	0.03
Baking powder, double-acting, sodium and aluminum (1 tsp.)	0	0	270	1	100	0
Baking powder, double-acting, straight phosphate (1 tsp.)	0	0	338	2	456	0

Spices

	VIT A (IU)	VIT C (mg)	CAL (mg)	MAG (mg)	PHOS (mg)	ZINC (mg)
Allspice, ground (1 tsp.)	10	1	13	3	2	0.02
Anise seed (1 tsp.)	7	0	14	4	9	0.11
Basil, fresh (2 tbsp.)	205	1	8	4	4	0.05
Basil, ground (1 tsp.)	131	1	30	6	7	0.08

	VIT A (IU)	VIT C (mg)	CAL (mg)	MAG (mg)	PHOS (mg)	ZINC (mg)
Bay leaf, crumbled (1 tsp.)	37	0	5	1	1	0.02
Caraway seed (1 tsp.)	8	0	15	5	12	0.12
Cardamon, ground (1 tsp.)	0	0	8	5	4	0.15
Celery seed (1 tsp.)	1	0	35	9	11	0.14
Chervil, dried (1 tsp.)	35	0	8	1	3	0.05
Chili powder (1 tsp.)	908	2	7	4	8	0.07
Cilantro (1 oz.)	256	3	*	*	*	*
Cinnamon, ground (1 tsp.)	6	1	28	1	1	0.05
Cloves, ground (1 tsp.)	11	2	14	6	2	0.02
Coriander leaf, dried (1 tsp.)	35	3	8	4	3	0.03
Coriander seed (1 tsp.)	0	0	13	6	7	0.09
Cumin seed (1 tsp.)	27	0	20	8	10	0.1
Curry powder (1 tsp.)	20	0	10	5	7	0.08
Dill seed (1 tsp.)	1	0	32	5	6	0.11
Dill weed, dried (1 tsp.)	59	1	18	5	5	0.03
Dill weed, fresh (10 sprigs)	144	2	5	1	1	0.02
Fennel seed (1 tsp.)	3	0	24	8	10	0.07
Fenugreek seed (1 tsp.)	2	0	7	7	11	0.09
Garlic powder (1 tsp.)	0	1	2	2	12	0.07
Ginger, ground (1 tsp.)	3	0	2	3	3	0.09
Mace, ground (1 tsp.)	14	0	4	3	2	0.04
Marjoram, dried (1 tsp.)	48	0	12	2	2	0.02
Mustard, seed, yellow (1 tsp.)	2	0	17	10	28	0.19
Nutmeg, ground (1 tsp.)	2	0	4	4	5	0.05
Onion powder (1 tsp.)	0	0	8	3	7	0.05
Oregano, ground (1 tsp.)	104	1	24	4	3	0.07
Parsley, dried (1 tsp.)	70	0	4	1	1	0.01
Pepper, black (1 tsp.)	4	0	9	4	4	0.03
Pepper, red or cayenne (1 tsp.)	749	1	3	3	5	0.05
Pepper, white (1 tsp.)	0	1	6	2	4	0.03
Poppy seed (1 tsp.)	0	0	41	9	24	0.29

	VIT A (IU)	VIT C (mg)	CAL (mg)	MAG (mg)	PHOS (mg)	ZINC (mg)
Poultry seasoning (1 tsp.)	40	0	15	3	3	0.05
Pumpkin pie spice (1 tsp.)	4	0	12	2	2	0.04
Rosemary, dried (1 tsp.)	38	1	15	3	1	0.04
Saffron (1 tsp.)	4	1	1	2	2	0.01
Sage, ground (1 tsp.)	41	0	12	3	1	0.03
Salt, table (1 tsp.)	0	0	1	0	0	0.01
Savory, ground (1 tsp.)	72	1	30	5	2	0.06
Thyme, fresh (1 tsp.)	38	1	3	1	1	0.01
Thyme, ground (1 tsp.)	53	1	26	3	3	0.09
Tumeric, ground (1 tsp.)	0	1	4	4	6	0.1

Sugars and syrups

	VIT A (IU)	VIT C (mg)	CAL (mg)	MAG (mg)	PHOS (mg)	ZINC (mg)
Sugar						
Brown (1 tsp.)	0	0	3	1	1	0.01
Granulated (1 tsp.)	0	0	0	0	0	0
Maple (1 oz.)	7	0	26	5	1	1.72
Powdered (1 tsp.)	0	0	0	0	0	0
Syrups						
Corn, dark (1 tbsp.)	0	0	4	2	2	0.01
Corn, table blends, refined and sugar (1 tbsp.)	0	0	5	2	2	0.01
Molasses, blackstrap (1 tbsp.)	0	0	172	43	8	0.02
Pancake, table blend (1 tbsp.)	0	0	0	0	2	0.01
Pancake, table blend, reduced-calorie (1 oz.)	0	0	0	0	12	0.01
Syrups, flavored						
Chocolate, with added nutrients, prepared with milk (1 cup)	1126	2	292	32	229	0.92
Strawberry-flavor beverage mix prepared with milk (1 cup)	309	2	293	32	229	0.93

Thickening Agent	VIT A (IU)	VIT C (mg)	CAL (mg)	MAG (mg)	PHOS (mg)	ZINC (mg)
Cornstarch (1 cup)	0	0	3	4	17	0.07

NUTS, SEEDS, AND BUTTERS

Nuts

	VIT A (IU)	VIT C (mg)	CAL (mg)	MAG (mg)	PHOS (mg)	ZINC (mg)
Almonds						
Honey roasted (1 oz.)	0	0	75	68	113	0.74
Dried, blanched (1 oz.)	0	0	70	81	151	0.9
Dry roasted, unblanched (1 oz.)	0	0	80	86	155	1.39
Oil roasted, blanched (1 oz.)	0	0	55	82	164	0.4
Toasted, unblanched (1 oz.)	0	0	80	87	156	1.4
Butternuts, dried (1 oz.)	35	1	15	67	126	0.89
Cashew nuts, dry-roasted (1 oz.)	0	0	13	74	139	1.59
Chestnuts, Chinese, roasted (1 oz.)	1	11	5	26	29	0.26
Coconut meat, raw, shredded (1 cup)	0	3	11	26	90	0.88
Filberts, dried, unblanched (1 oz.)	19	0	53	81	89	0.68
Filberts, dry-roasted, unblanched (1 oz.)	0	0	55	84	92	0.71
Ginkgo, canned (1 oz.)	96	3	1	5	15	0.06
Ginkgo, dried (1 oz.)	309	8	6	15	76	0.19
Macadamia, dried (1 oz.)	0	0	20	33	39	0.49
Macadamia, oil-roasted (1 oz.)	3	0	13	33	57	0.31
Mixed nuts, dry-roasted, with peanuts (1 oz.)	4	0	20	64	123	1.08
Peanuts, all types, raw (1 oz.)	0	0	26	48	107	0.93
Pecans, dried (1 oz.)	36	1	10	36	83	1.55
Pine, dried (10 kernels)	0	0	0	2	0	0.04
Pine, pignolia, dried (1 oz.)	8	1	7	66	144	1.21
Pistachio, dried (1 oz.)	66	2	38	45	143	0.38

	VIT A (IU)	VIT C (mg)	CAL (mg)	MAG (mg)	PHOS (mg)	ZINC (mg)
Pistachio, dry-roasted (1 oz.)	67	2	20	37	135	0.39
Soy, roasted (1 oz.)	0	0	60	*	*	*
Walnuts, black, dried (1 oz.)	84	1	16	57	132	0.97
Walnuts, English or Persian, dried (1 oz.)	35	1	27	48	90	0.77
Wheat based, unflavored (1 oz.)	0	0	7	16	105	0.83

Seeds

	VIT A (IU)	VIT C (mg)	CAL (mg)	MAG (mg)	PHOS (mg)	ZINC (mg)
Alfalfa, sprouted, raw (1 cup)	51	3	11	9	23	0.3
Breadfruit, boiled (1 oz.)	68	2	17	4	35	0.24
Breadfruit, raw (1 oz.)	73	2	10	15	50	0.27
Breadnut tree seeds, dried (1 oz.)	61	13	27	33	51	0.54
Breadnut tree seeds, raw (1 oz., 8–14 seeds)	70	8	28	19	19	0.32
Pumpkin kernels, roasted (1 oz.)	108	1	12	152	333	2.11
Pumpkin and squash seed kernels, roasted, with salt (1 oz.)	108	1	12	152	333	2.11
Pumpkin and squash seed kernels, roasted, with salt (1 cup)	862	4	98	1212	2660	16.9
Sesame, whole, dried (1 tbsp.)	1	0	88	32	57	0.7
Sesame, whole, roasted and toasted (1 oz.)	3	0	280	101	181	2.03
Soybeans, mature, roasted (½ cup)	172	2	119	125	312	2.7
Squash, kernels, roasted (1 oz.)	108	1	12	151	332	2.11

	VIT A (IU)	VIT C (mg)	CAL (mg)	MAG (mg)	PHOS (mg)	ZINC (mg)
Sunflower seeds						
Dried (1/2 cup)	36	1	134	255	507	3.6
Dry-roasted (1 oz.)	0	0	20	37	327	1.5
Roasted (1/2 cup)	*	*	40	220	500	*
Roasted, reduced-sodium (1/2 cup)	*	*	40	220	500	*
Roasted, reduced-sodium (1 cup)	*	*	80	440	1000	*
Watermelon kernels, dried (1 oz.)	0	0	15	146	214	2.9

Butters

	VIT A (IU)	VIT C (mg)	CAL (mg)	MAG (mg)	PHOS (mg)	ZINC (mg)
Almond, honey and cinnamon (1 tbsp.)	0	0	43	48	83	0.48
Almond, plain (1 tbsp.)	0	0	43	49	84	0.49
Almond paste (1 oz.)	0	<1	65	73	127	0.73
Apple butter (1 tbsp.)	0	*	1	0	1	0.01
Cashew, plain (1 tbsp.)	0	0	7	41	73	0.83
Peanut, chunk style (2 tbsp.)	0	0	13	51	101	0.89
Peanut, Plus Vitamins and Minerals (2 tbsp.)	1250	*	*	87	*	3
Peanut, reduced-fat (2 tbsp.)	0	0	0	45	0	0.9
Peanut, smooth style (2 tbsp.)	0	0	12	51	118	0.93
Sesame, paste (1 tbsp.)	8	0	154	58	105	1.17
Sesame, tahini, from roasted and toasted kernels (1 tbsp.)	10	0	64	14	110	0.69
Sunflower seed (1 tbsp.)	8	0	20	59	118	0.85

PASTA, NOODLES, AND RICE

Pasta

	VIT A (IU)	VIT C (mg)	CAL (mg)	MAG (mg)	PHOS (mg)	ZINC (mg)
Corn, cooked (1 cup)	80	0	1	50	106	0.88

	VIT A (IU)	VIT C (mg)	CAL (mg)	MAG (mg)	PHOS (mg)	ZINC (mg)
Corn, dry (2 oz.)	97	0	2	68	144	1.02
Couscous, cooked (1 cup)	0	0	13	13	35	0.41
Homemade, with egg, cooked (2 oz.)	33	0	6	8	30	0.25
Homemade, without egg, cooked (2 oz.)	0	0	3	8	23	0.21
Plain, fresh-refrigerated, as purchased (4.5 oz.)	60	0	19	59	209	1.56
Plain, fresh-refrigerated, cooked (2 oz.)	11	0	3	10	36	0.32
Spaghetti						
Protein-fortified, dry pasta, enriched (2 oz.)	0	0	22	37	93	1.02
Spinach pasta, cooked (1 cup)	213	0	42	87	151	1.51
Spinach, fresh-refrigerated, as purchased (4.5 oz.)	308	0	55	81	189	1.79
Spinach pasta, fresh-refrigerated, cooked (2 oz.)	59	0	10	14	33	0.36
Whole wheat, dry pasta (2 oz.)	0	0	23	82	147	1.35

Noodles

	VIT A (IU)	VIT C (mg)	CAL (mg)	MAG (mg)	PHOS (mg)	ZINC (mg)
Chinese, chow mein (1.5 oz.)	37	0	9	22	69	0.6
Egg, enriched, cooked (1 cup)	32	0	19	30	110	0.99
Egg, spinach, enriched, cooked (1 cup)	165	0	30	38	91	1.01

	VIT A (IU)	VIT C (mg)	CAL (mg)	MAG (mg)	PHOS (mg)	ZINC (mg)
Macaroni, protein-fortified, enriched, cooked (½ cup)	0	0	6	17	29	0.29
Macaroni, vegetable, enriched, cooked (1 cup)	71	0	15	26	67	0.59
Macaroni, whole-wheat, dry (1 cup)	0	0	42	150	271	2.49
Protein-fortified, enriched, dry (2 oz.)	0	0	22	37	93	1.02
Soba, Japanese, cooked (1 cup)	0	0	5	10	29	0.14
Somen, Japanese, cooked (1 cup)	0	0	14	4	48	0.39
Whole wheat, elbow, dry (1 cup)	0	0	23	82	147	1.35
Whole wheat, spiral, dry (1 cup)	0	0	42	150	271	2.49

Rice *(see also* Grains)

	VIT A (IU)	VIT C (mg)	CAL (mg)	MAG (mg)	PHOS (mg)	ZINC (mg)
Brown, long-grained, cooked (1 cup)	0	0	20	84	162	1.23
White, glutinous, cooked (1 cup)	0	0	4	9	14	0.71
White, long-grained, parboiled, enriched, cooked (1 cup)	0	0	33	21	74	0.54
White, long-grained, precooked or instant, enriched, prepared (1 cup)	0	0	13	8	23	0.4
White, long-grained, regular, cooked (1 cup)	0	0	16	19	68	0.77
White, with pasta, cooked (1 cup)	0	0	16	24	75	0.57

	VIT A (IU)	VIT C (mg)	CAL (mg)	MAG (mg)	PHOS (mg)	ZINC (mg)
White, with pasta, dry (1 cup)	0	1	75	65	258	1.97
Wild, cooked (1 cup)	0	0	5	53	135	2.2

POULTRY

Chicken

	VIT A (IU)	VIT C (mg)	CAL (mg)	MAG (mg)	PHOS (mg)	ZINC (mg)
Broilers or fryers, fried						
Breast, meat and skin, floured, bone removed (½ breast)	49	0	16	29	228	1.08
Dark meat, meat only (1 cup)	111	0	25	35	262	4.08
Giblets (1 cup)	17,297	13	26	36	415	0.09
Light meat, meat only (1 cup)	42	0	22	41	323	1.78
Broilers or fryers, roasted						
Back, meat only, bone and skin removed (½ back)	38	0	10	9	66	1.06
Breast, meat and skin, bone removed (½ breast)	91	0	14	27	210	1
Breast, meat only, bone and skin removed (½ breast)	18	0	13	25	196	0.86
Dark meat, meat and skin, ready to cook chicken (1 lb.)	203	0	15	22	170	2.52
Dark meat, meat only (1 cup, chopped)	101	0	21	32	251	3.92
Drumstick, meat only, bone and skin removed (1 drumstick)	26	0	5	11	81	1.4

	VIT A (IU)	VIT C (mg)	CAL (mg)	MAG (mg)	PHOS (mg)	ZINC (mg)
Light meat, meat only, chopped (1 cup)	41	0	21	38	302	1.72
Light meat, meat and skin, ready-to-cook (1 lb.)	87	0	12	20	158	0.97
Meat, skin, giblets, and neck, ready-to-cook (1 lb.)	1304	1	31	47	373	4.43
Thigh, meat only (1 cup)	91	0	17	34	256	3.6
Cornish game hens, meat and skin (½ bird)	136	0.5	17	23	188	1.92
Cornish game hens, meat and skin (1 whole bird)	272	1	33	46	375	3.83
Frankfurter, chicken (1 frankfurter)	59	0	43	5	48	0.47
Liver, all classes, simmered (1 cup, chopped)	22,925	22	20	29	437	6.08

Meatless Poultry

	VIT A (IU)	VIT C (mg)	CAL (mg)	MAG (mg)	PHOS (mg)	ZINC (mg)
Chicken, vegetarian, canned, Worthington (3 slices)	0	0	13	*	112	0.4
Chicken, vegetarian, frozen, Morningstar Farms (1 patty)	0	0	11	*	121	0.31
Chicken Nuggets, vegetarian, Loma Linda (5 pieces)	0	0	41	*	*	0.43

Turkey	VIT A (IU)	VIT C (mg)	CAL (mg)	MAG (mg)	PHOS (mg)	ZINC (mg)
Bologna (2 slices)	0	0	48	8	74	0.99
Breast (2 slices)	0	0	3	9	97	0.48
Breast, meat and skin, ready-to-cook (1 lb.)	0	0	24	30	235	2.27
Dark meat (1 cup, chopped)	0	0	45	34	286	6.24
Frankfurter, turkey (1 frankfurter)	0	0	48	6	60	1.4
Giblets, simmered (1 cup, chopped)	8752	3	19	25	296	5.34
Gizzard, simmered (1 cup, cooked)	268	2	22	28	186	6.03
Ground, cooked (1 patty, 4 oz. raw)	0	0	21	20	161	2.35
Ham, cured turkey thigh meat (2 slices)	0	0	6	9	108	1.67
Hen, young, meat only, roasted (1 cup, chopped)	0	0	35	36	297	4.24
Leg, meat and skin, roasted, bone removed (1 leg)	0	0	175	126	1087	23.31
Liver, simmered (1 cup, chopped)	17,613	3	15	21	381	4.33
Meat only, roasted (1 cup, chopped)	0	0	35	36	298	4.34
Meat, skin, giblets, and neck, roasted, ready to cook (1 lb.)	598	0	68	62	520	8.19
Pastrami, turkey (2 slices)	0	0	5	8	113	1.23
Patties, turkey, breaded, battered, fried (1 patty)	35	0	13	14	254	1.35
Roll, turkey, light meat (2 slices)	0	0	23	9	104	0.89
Roll, turkey, dark meat (2 slices)	0	0	18	10	95	1.13

	VIT A (IU)	VIT C (mg)	CAL (mg)	MAG (mg)	PHOS (mg)	ZINC (mg)
Salami, cooked, turkey (2 slices)	0	0	11	9	60	1.03

Game and Other Poultry

Duck

	VIT A (IU)	VIT C (mg)	CAL (mg)	MAG (mg)	PHOS (mg)	ZINC (mg)
Domesticated, meat only, roasted, ready-to-cook (1 lb.)	77	0	12	20	203	2.6
Domesticated, meat and skin, roasted, ready-to-cook (1 lb.)	363	0	19	28	270	3.22
Wild, breast, meat only, raw, skin removed (½ breast)	44	5	3	18	154	0.61

Goose

	VIT A (IU)	VIT C (mg)	CAL (mg)	MAG (mg)	PHOS (mg)	ZINC (mg)
Domesticated, meat only, roasted, ready-to-cook (1 lb.)	57	0	20	36	442	4.53
Domesticated, meat and skin, roasted, ready-to-cook (1 lb.)	132	0	24	41	508	4.93
Pâté, goose liver, smoked, canned (1 oz.)	945	0	20	4	57	0.26

Pheasant

	VIT A (IU)	VIT C (mg)	CAL (mg)	MAG (mg)	PHOS (mg)	ZINC (mg)
Breast, meat only, raw, bone and skin removed (½ breast)	268	11	6	38	364	1.15
Meat only, raw, ready-to-cook (1 lb.)	538	20	42	65	750	3.16
Meat and skin, raw, ready-to-cook (1 lb.)	657	20	45	74	794	3.56

	VIT A (IU)	VIT C (mg)	CAL (mg)	MAG (mg)	PHOS (mg)	ZINC (mg)
Quail, meat and skin, raw (1 oz.)	69	2	4	*	61	*

PREPARED FOODS

	VIT A (IU)	VIT C (mg)	CAL (mg)	MAG (mg)	PHOS (mg)	ZINC (mg)
Amaranth Dinner with Garden Vegetables, canned, Health Valley (7½ oz.)	*	*	40	*	*	*
Beans						
Plain or vegetarian (1 cup)	434	8	127	81	264	3.56
With franks, canned (1 cup)	399	6	124	73	269	4.84
With franks, frozen, Banquet (10¼ oz.)	4450	*	130	*	*	*
Baked, with pork and sweet sauce, canned (1 cup)	288	8	154	86	266	3.8
Baked, with pork and sweet sauce, canned (1 cup)	288	8	154	86	266	3.8
Beef, Extra Helping, frozen, Banquet (10¼ oz.)	4600	*	80	*	*	*
Biscuit, Egg and Cheese, frozen, precooked, Sunny Fresh (1 serving)	205	0	101	3	50	0.3
Biscuit, egg and steak (1 biscuit)	705	0	138	25	225	2.8
Biscuit, Egg, Ham and Cheese, Sunny Fresh (1 serving)	213	0	106	4	54	0.33
Black Bean Dinner, with Garden Vegetables, Health Valley (7½ oz.)	4550	*	150	*	*	0.96
Brunswick Stew, homemade (1 cup)	400	*	30	*	*	1.67

	VIT A (IU)	VIT C (mg)	CAL (mg)	MAG (mg)	PHOS (mg)	ZINC (mg)
Chicken and Dumplings, frozen, Banquet (9 oz.)	2950	*	50	*	*	*
Chicken in Cheese Sauce with Broccoli, frozen, Light and Elegant (8¾ oz.)	350	*	170	*	*	*
Chicken Piccatta with Rice, frozen, Prego (11 oz.)	850	*	80	*	*	*
Chicken with Broccoli, frozen, Light and Elegant (9½ oz.)	350	*	170	*	*	*
Chopped Beef, frozen, Banquet (11 oz.)	6400	*	60	*	*	*
Chili, Beans, Nestlé, Chef-Mate (1 cup)	3013	1	89	46	167	3.87
Chili, beans, canned (1 cup)	863	4	120	115	394	5.12
Corn pudding (⅔ cup)	411	5	67	25	95	0.84
Enchilada Beef, frozen, Banquet (12 oz.)	350	*	170	*	*	*
Enchilada, cheese (1 enchilada)	300	9	150	*	*	*
Enchilada, black bean, vegetable (1 enchilada)	400	6	40	*	*	*
Garden Vegetable Lasagna, Campbell's, frozen (1 cup)	3500	3	450	*	*	*
Hash, corned beef (1 cup)	0	2	46	38	240	7.51
Hush puppy, prepared from recipe (1 hush puppy)	31	0	61	5	42	0.15
Hummus (1 cup)	61	19	124	71	275	2.7

	VIT A (IU)	VIT C (mg)	CAL (mg)	MAG (mg)	PHOS (mg)	ZINC (mg)
Lasagna Alfredo, Weight Watcher's (½ cup)	200	6	250	*	*	*
Florentine, frozen, Light and Elegant (12 oz.)	1300	*	70	*	*	*
Meat Sauce, frozen, Banquet (11¼ oz.)	3850	*	230	*	*	*
Lentil Dinner, with Garden Vegetable, canned, Health Valley (7½ oz.)	5200	*	70	*	*	0.64
Macaroni and cheese						
Canned, Franco-American (7½ oz.)	550	*	170	*	*	*
Kraft (¾ cup)	350	*	100	*	*	1.28
Nestlé, Chef-Mate (1 cup)	210	0	202	33	251	1.57
Manicotti with 3 Cheeses, Healthy Choice, frozen (1 serving)	750	*	350	*	*	*
Mexican Style Dinner, Extra Helping, Banquet (21¼ oz.)	1200	*	340	*	*	*
Muffins, wheat bran, prepared from recipe, with whole milk (1 muffin)	459	5	106	45	163	1.57
Onion rings, breaded, frozen (7 rings)	158	1	22	13	57	0.29
Pasta Primavera Style, frozen, Bird's Eye (½ cup)	4050	*	80	*	*	0.64
Peas and Potatoes with Cream Sauce, Bird's Eye (½ cup)	500	*	40	*	*	0.48
Pizza, cheese (1 slice)	382	1	117	16	113	0.81
Pizza, cheese, meat, and vegetables (1 slice)	524	2	101	18	131	1.11

	VIT A (IU)	VIT C (mg)	CAL (mg)	MAG (mg)	PHOS (mg)	ZINC (mg)
Pizza sauce, ready-to-serve (¼ cup)	420	7	34	13	32	0.16
Poi, taro root (1 cup)	48	10	38	58	94	0.53
Potatoes						
Au gratin, dry mix, prepared with water, whole milk, and butter (⅙ of 5.5 oz. package)	292	4	114	21	130	0.33
Au gratin, home-prepared from recipe using butter (1 cup)	647	24	292	49	277	1.69
Cream and Chives, baked, frozen, Pillsbury (1 potato)	400	*	40	*	*	*
French fried, home-prepared, heated in oven (10 strips)	0	5	4	11	41	0.2
Hash brown, frozen, butter sauce, prepared (100 g)	111	4	33	15	38	0.33
Hash brown, frozen, plain, prepared (1 oval patty)	0	2	4	5	21	0.09
Hash brown, home-prepared (1 cup)	0	9	13	31	66	0.47
Mashed, dehydrated, granules with milk, dry form (1 cup)	120	32	284	148	474	2.4
Mashed, flakes, without milk, dry (1 cup)	0	40	12	31	74	0.33
Mashed, home-prepared, whole milk and margarine added (1 cup)	355	13	55	38	97	0.57

	VIT A (IU)	VIT C (mg)	CAL (mg)	MAG (mg)	PHOS (mg)	ZINC (mg)
Mashed, home-prepared, whole milk, butter (1 cup)	355	13	55	38	97	0.57
Potato pancakes, home-prepared (1 pancake)	109	17	18	25	84	0.63
Potato salad (1/3 cup)	95	1	13	8	53	0.19
Scalloped, dry mix, prepared with water, whole milk, and butter (1/6 of 5.5 oz. package)	203	5	49	19	77	0.34
Scalloped, home-prepared with butter (1/2 cup)	166	13	70	24	77	0.49
Scalloped, home-prepared with butter (1 cup)	331	26	140	47	154	0.98
Ravioli with Meat, Sausage and Peppers, Prego Plus (1 cup)	2000	*	80	*	*	*
Refried beans, canned (1/2 cup)	*	8	44	42	109	1.48
Refried beans, canned (1 cup)	*	15	88	83	217	2.95
Relish, cranberry-orange, canned (1/2 cup)	87	25	15	11	11	*
Relish, cranberry-orange, canned (1 cup)	193	50	30	11	22	*
Rice						
Black-Eyed Peas and Rice, Zatarain, prepared (1/2 cup)	*	0	40	*	*	*
Dirty Rice Mix, Zatarain, prepared (1 cup)	100	1	40	*	*	*

	VIT A (IU)	VIT C (mg)	CAL (mg)	MAG (mg)	PHOS (mg)	ZINC (mg)
Pinto Beans and Rice, Uncle Ben's, prepared (1 cup)	400	3	40	*	*	*
Wild Rice & Mushroom Stuffing Mix, Pepperidge Farm, prepared (⅔ cup)	*	6	40	*	*	*
Rosetto, cheese stuffed shells (2 pieces)	400	*	200	*	*	*
Shrimp Creole, with Rice and Peppers, Light and Elegant (10 oz.)	2200	*	60	*	*	*
Spaghetti with Meat Sauce, canned, Prego (12½ oz.)	1300	*	40	*	*	*
Spanish Rice, canned, Van Camp (1 cup)	1150	*	30	*	*	*
Spinach soufflé (1 cup)	3461	3	230	38	231	1.29
Stew, Beef, Nestlé, Chef-Mate (1 cup)	3107	3	63	35	159	2.5
Stuffing, corn bread, prepared (½ cup)	44	1	22	12	32	0.21
Stuffing, prepared (½ cup)	*	*	28	11	40	0.26
Tomato Pasta Florentine, frozen, Campbell's (½ cup)	750	6	80	*	*	*
Tuna Pot Pie, frozen, Banquet (1 cup)	150	*	50	*	*	*
Turkey Pot Pie, frozen, Banquet (1 cup)	150	*	40	*	*	*
Turkey Tetrazzini, frozen, Banquet (10 oz.)	350	*	120	*	*	*

	VIT A (IU)	VIT C (mg)	CAL (mg)	MAG (mg)	PHOS (mg)	ZINC (mg)
Veal Parmigiana, frozen, Banquet (11 oz.)	750	*	100	*	*	*
Taco mix (3 tbsp.)	122	0	29	*	*	0.32

Vegetarian Entrées

	VIT A (IU)	VIT C (mg)	CAL (mg)	MAG (mg)	PHOS (mg)	ZINC (mg)
Beans, plain or vegetarian (1 cup)	434	8	127	81	264	3.56
Burgers						
Black Bean Burgers, spicy, Morningstar Farms (1 patty)	0	0	40	*	*	*
California Veggie Burger, Organic Vegetables, Amy's (1 burger)	1500	3	20	*	*	*
Garden Vege Patties, Morningstar Farms (1 patty)	3	0	40	*	*	*
Egg Roll, Vegetarian, frozen, Worthington (3 oz. roll)	0	0	15	*	70	0.31
Falafel (2¼" patty)	2	*	9	14	33	0.26
Hummus, commercially prepared (½ cup)	31	10	62	36	138	1.35
Hummus, prepared from recipe (1 cup)	61	19	124	71	275	2.7
Lentil-Rice Loaf, Natural Touch (3.2 oz. slice)	775	0	21	*	213	1.04
Nine-Bean Loaf, Natural Touch (1" slice, 3 oz.)	1509	1	27	*	*	0.88
Savory Dinner Loaf, Loma Linda (⅓ cup)	0	0	23	*	*	0.38
Spinach Feta Pocketfuls, Amy's (1 serving)	2250	5	250	*	*	*

	VIT A (IU)	VIT C (mg)	CAL (mg)	MAG (mg)	PHOS (mg)	ZINC (mg)
Tempeh (½ cup)	569	0	77	58	171	1.5
Vegetable Lasagna, Amy's (1 container)	2500	21	200	*	*	*
Vegetable Pot Pie, Amy's (1 container)	2250	5	100	*	*	*
Veggie Loaf, Mashed potatoes and Vegetables, Amy's (1 container)	2250	36	40	*	*	*

SALADS

	VIT A (IU)	VIT C (mg)	CAL (mg)	MAG (mg)	PHOS (mg)	ZINC (mg)
Coleslaw (¾ cup)	338	8	34	9	36	0.2
Crab (1 serving)	30	2	38	26	*	*
Chef (1 serving)	2997	21	150	*	*	*
Carrot and raisin, homemade (1 serving)	3663	12	96	42	*	*
Tuna, with bread, lettuce, and oil (9 oz.)	188	4	74	79	219	*
Vegetable salads						
With egg and cheese, without dressing (1½ cups)	822	10	100	24	132	1
With chicken, without dressing (1½ cups)	935	17	37	33	170	0.89
With shrimp, without dressing (1½ cups)	791	9	59	38	161	1.27
Without dressing (1½ cups)	2352	48	27	23	81	0.44
Potato, homemade (1 cup)	500	*	40	*	*	0.61
Taco (1½ cups)	588	4	192	52	143	2.69
Taboule wheat salad mix (1 tbsp.)	100	0	40	*	*	*

SALAD DRESSINGS	VIT A (IU)	VIT C (mg)	CAL (mg)	MAG (mg)	PHOS (mg)	ZINC (mg)
Blue or Roquefort cheese, regular (1 tbsp.)	32	0	12	0	11	0.04
French, diet, low-fat, 5 calories per teaspoon (1 tbsp.)	212	0	2	0	2	0.03
French, regular (1 tbsp.)	203	0	2	0	2	0.01
Italian, diet, 2 calories per teaspoon (1 tbsp.)	0	0	0	0	1	0.02
Italian, diet, commercial (packet)	0	0	1	0	3	0.07
Italian, regular (1 tbsp.)	12	0	2	0	1	0.02
Oil and Vinegar, prepared by recipe (1 tbsp.)	0	0	0	0	*	*
Sesame seed (1 tbsp.)	106	0	3	0	6	0.02
Russian (1 tbsp.)	106	1	3	0	6	0.07
Thousand island, commercial (1 tbsp.)	50	0	2	0	3	0.02
Thousand island, diet, 10 calories per teaspoon (1 tbsp.)	49	0	2	0	3	0.02
Thousand island, regular (1 tbsp.)	50	0	2	0	3	0.02

SEAFOOD

	VIT A (IU)	VIT C (mg)	CAL (mg)	MAG (mg)	PHOS (mg)	ZINC (mg)
Anchovy, European, canned in oil, drained (1 can, 2 oz.)	32	0	104	31	113	1.1
Anchovy, European, raw (3 oz.)	43	0	125	35	148	1.46
Bass, fresh water, mixed species, cooked, dry heat (3 oz.)	98	2	88	32	218	0.71
Bass, fresh water, mixed species, raw (3 oz.)	85	2	68	26	170	0.55

	VIT A (IU)	VIT C (mg)	CAL (mg)	MAG (mg)	PHOS (mg)	ZINC (mg)
Bluefish, cooked, dry heat (3 oz.)	390	0	8	36	247	0.88
Burbot, cooked, dry heat (3 oz.)	15	0	54	35	218	0.83
Butterfish, cooked, dry heat (3 oz.)	93	0	24	27	262	0.84
Catfish, channel, breaded, fried (1 fillet)	24	0	38	24	188	0.75
Catfish, channel, farmed, cooked, dry heat (3 oz.)	43	1	8	22	208	0.89
Catfish, channel, wild, cooked, dry heat (3 oz.)	43	1	9	24	258	0.52
Caviar, black and red, granular (1 oz.)	530	0	78	85	101	0.27
Clam, mixed species, canned, drained solids (3 oz.)	485	19	78	15	287	2.32
Clam, mixed species, breaded and fried (3 oz.)	257	9	54	12	160	1.24
Cod, Atlantic, cooked, dry heat (1 fillet)	83	2	25	76	248	1.04
Cod liver oil (1 tbsp.)	13,600	0	0	0	0	0
Crab						
Alaska king, cooked, moist heat (3 oz.)	25	7	50	54	238	6.48
Alaska king, imitation, made from surimi (3 oz.)	56	0	11	37	240	0.28
Baked (1 crab)	77	3	415	82	337	7.02
Cake (1 cake)	313	0	202	25	227	2.12
Blue, canned (3 oz.)	4	2	86	33	221	3.42
Dungeness, cooked, moist heat (1 crab)	132	5	75	74	222	6.95

	VIT A (IU)	VIT C (mg)	CAL (mg)	MAG (mg)	PHOS (mg)	ZINC (mg)
Soft-shell, fried (1 crab)	15	1	55	25	131	1.06
Crayfish, mixed species, farmed, cooked, moist heat (3 oz.)	43	0	43	28	205	1.26
Cod, Pacific, cooked, dry heat (3 oz.)	27	3	8	26	190	0.43
Dolphinfish, cooked, dry heat (3 oz.)	177	0	16	32	156	0.5
Fish fillet, battered or breaded, and fried (1 fillet)	35	0	16	22	156	0.4
Fish sticks, breaded, frozen (1 oz.)	30	*	6	7	51	0.19
Grouper, mixed species, cooked, dry heat (1 fillet)	333	0	42	75	289	1.03
Halibut, Greenland, cooked, dry heat (3 oz.)	51	0	3	28	179	0.43
Lobster, Northern, cooked, moist heat (3 oz.)	74	0	52	30	157	2.48
Lobster, spiny, mixed species, cooked, moist heat (3 oz.)	17	2	54	43	195	6.18
Herring, Atlantic, cooked, dry heat (3 oz.)	87	1	63	35	258	1.08
Herring, Atlantic, kippered (1 oz.)	36	0	24	13	92	0.39
Herring, Pacific, cooked, dry heat (3 oz.)	99	0	90	35	248	0.58
Mackerel, king, cooked, dry heat (3 oz.)	713	1	34	35	270	0.61
Monkfish, cooked, dry heat (3 oz.)	39	1	9	23	218	0.45

	VIT A (IU)	VIT C (mg)	CAL (mg)	MAG (mg)	PHOS (mg)	ZINC (mg)
Ocean perch, Atlantic, cooked, dry heat (3 oz.)	39	1	117	33	236	0.52
Oyster, Eastern, canned (3 oz.)	255	4	38	46	118	77.31
Perch, mixed species, cooked, dry heat (3 oz.)	27	2	87	32	219	1.22
Pompano, Florida, cooked, dry heat (1 fillet)	106	0	38	27	300	0.61
Red snapper, cooked, dry heat (3 oz.)	326	1	34	31	*	*
Rockfish, cooked, dry heat (3 oz.)	326	1	10	29	*	*
Roe, mixed species, cooked, dry heat (3 oz.)	258	14	24	22	438	1.09
Roughy, orange, cooked, dry heat (3 oz.)	69	0	32	32	218	0.82
Roughy, orange, raw (3 oz.)	60	0	26	26	170	0.64
Salmon, Atlantic, farmed, cooked, dry heat (3 oz.)	43	3	13	26	214	0.37
Salmon, Atlantic, wild, cooked, dry heat (3 oz.)	37	0	13	32	218	0.7
Salmon, chinook, cooked, dry heat (3 oz.)	422	4	24	104	315	0.48
Salmon, chinook, smoked (3 oz.)	75	0	9	15	139	0.26
Salmon, chum, drained solids with bone and liquid (3 oz.)	52	0	212	26	301	0.85
Salmon, pink, canned, solids with bone and liquid (3 oz.)	47	0	181	29	280	0.78

	VIT A (IU)	VIT C (mg)	CAL (mg)	MAG (mg)	PHOS (mg)	ZINC (mg)
Salmon, pink, cooked, dry heat (3 oz.)	116	0	15	28	251	0.6
Sardines, Atlantic, canned in oil, drained solids with bone (3.75 oz.)	206	0	351	36	451	1.21
Sardines, fish oil (1 tbsp.)	0	0	0	0	0	0
Sardines, Pacific, canned in tomato sauce, drained solids with bone (1 cup)	325	1	214	30	326	1.25
Scallop, mixed species, breaded and fried (2 large scallops)	23	1	13	18	73	0.33
Sea bass, mixed species, cooked, dry heat (3 oz.)	181	0	11	45	211	0.44
Sea trout, mixed species, cooked, dry heat (3 oz.)	98	0	19	34	273	0.49
Sea trout, mixed species, raw (3 oz.)	85	0	15	26	213	0.38
Shad, American, cooked, dry heat (3 oz.)	102	0	51	32	297	0.4
Shark fin, prepared (1 cup)	0	0	22	15	45	1.77
Shark, mixed species, batter-dipped and fried (3 oz.)	153	0	43	37	165	0.41
Shark, mixed species, raw (100 g)	233	0	34	49	210	0.43
Shrimp, mixed species, canned (3 oz.)	51	2	50	35	198	1.07
Shrimp, mixed species, breaded and fried (3 oz.)	161	1	57	34	185	1.17

	VIT A (IU)	VIT C (mg)	CAL (mg)	MAG (mg)	PHOS (mg)	ZINC (mg)
Shrimp, mixed species, cooked, moist heat (3 oz.)	186	2	33	29	117	1.33
Snapper, mixed species, cooked, dry heat (3 oz.)	98	1	34	32	171	0.37
Sturgeon, cooked, dry heat (3 oz.)	*	*	11	30	*	*
Surimi, imitation crab and lobster (3 oz.)	57	*	8	37	*	*
Sunfish, pumpkin-seed, cooked, dry heat (3 oz.)	49	1	88	32	196	1.69
Swordfish, cooked, dry heat (3 oz.)	117	1	5	29	287	1.25
Trout, mixed species, cooked, dry heat (3 oz.)	54	0	47	24	267	0.72
Trout, rainbow, farmed, cooked, dry heat (3 oz.)	244	3	73	27	226	0.42
Tuna, light, canned in oil, drained, solids (3 oz.)	66	0	11	26	264	0.77
Tuna, light, canned in water, drained, solids (3 oz.)	48	0	9	23	139	0.66
Tuna, white, canned in oil, drained, solids (3 oz.)	68	0	3	29	227	0.4
Tuna, white, canned in water, drained solids (3 oz.)	16	0	12	28	185	0.41
Tuna, yellowfin, fresh, cooked, dry heat (3 oz.)	58	1	18	54	208	0.57
Turbot, European, cooked, dry heat (3 oz.)	34	2	20	55	140	0.24

	VIT A (IU)	VIT C (mg)	CAL (mg)	MAG (mg)	PHOS (mg)	ZINC (mg)
Yellowtail, mixed species, cooked, dry heat (3 oz.)	88	3	25	32	171	0.57
White perch, filet, fried (3 oz.)	8	*	12	*	*	*
Whitefish, mixed species, cooked, dry heat (3 oz.)	111	0	28	36	294	1.08
Whitefish, mixed species, smoked (3 oz.)	162	0	15	20	112	0.42
Vegetarian, tuna, Worthington (½ cup)	0	0	20	*	88	0.4

SNACK FOODS

	VIT A (IU)	VIT C (mg)	CAL (mg)	MAG (mg)	PHOS (mg)	ZINC (mg)
Banana chips (3 oz.)	71	5	15	65	48	0.64
Beef jerky, chopped and formed (1 oz.)	0	0	6	15	115	2.3
Chex mix (1 oz., approx. ⅔ cup)	41	14	10	18	53	0.59
Combos, Cheddar Cheese Pretzel (10 Combos)	20	0	59	7	43	0.22
Corn chips, barbecue-flavor (7 oz.)	1210	3	259	153	410	2.1
Corn chips, plain (7 oz.)	186	0	252	151	366	2.5
Corn puffs, cheese-flavor (1 oz.)	75	0	16	5	31	0.11
Corn twists, cheese-flavor (1 cup)	602	1	132	41	245	0.86
Cornnuts						
Barbecue-flavor (1 oz.)	96	0	5	31	80	0.53
Nacho-flavor (1 oz.)	11	4	10	31	88	0.51
Plain (1 oz.)	0	0	3	32	78	0.51
Doo Dads snack mix, original flavor (½ cup)	43	0	21	17	84	0.64

	VIT A (IU)	VIT C (mg)	CAL (mg)	MAG (mg)	PHOS (mg)	ZINC (mg)
Doughnuts, cake-type, plain, glazed or sugared (1 medium doughnut)	5	0	27	8	53	0.2
Ice cream cones, cake, wafer-type (1 cone)	0	0	1	1	4	0.03
Ice cream cones, sugar, rolled-type (1 cone)	0	.0	4	3	10	0.08
Oriental mix, rice-based (1 oz.)	1	0	15	34	74	0.75
Sesame sticks, wheat-based, salted (1 oz.)	25	0	48	13	39	0.33
Sweet Potato Chips, Terra Chips, Dana Alexander Inc. (1 oz.)	4000	0	20	*	*	*
Tortilla chips, nacho flavor (1 cup)	842	4	334	186	554	2.72
Tortilla chips, plain (7½ oz. bag)	418	0	328	187	437	3.26
Trail mix, regular (1 cup)	27	2	117	237	518	4.83
Trail mix, regular, with chocolate chips, salted nuts, and seeds (1 oz.)	13	0	31	46	110	0.89
Trail mix, tropical (1 oz.)	14	2	16	27	53	0.33
Tortilla chips, plain (1 oz.)	56	0	44	25	58	0.43

Frozen snacks (see also Desserts)

	VIT A (IU)	VIT C (mg)	CAL (mg)	MAG (mg)	PHOS (mg)	ZINC (mg)
Fruit Juice bars, grape, (1 bar)	0	18	0	0	0	0
Fruit leather bars, with cream (1 bar)	13	15	5	3	7	0.04
Ice Cream						
Chocolate (½ cup)	275	1	72	19	71	0.38
Chocolate, low-fat (½ cup)	270	*	85	9	69	0.45

	VIT A (IU)	VIT C (mg)	CAL (mg)	MAG (mg)	PHOS (mg)	ZINC (mg)
Vanilla (1/2 cup)	270	0	85	9	69	0.46
Ice milk, vanilla, soft-serve (1/2 cup)	91	1	138	12	107	0.05
Italian ice, (1/2 cup)	194	1	1	0	0	0.04
Sherbet, lemon (1/2 cup)	87	8	40	*	*	*
Sorbet, orange (1 cup)	70	6	60	*	*	*
Yogurt, vanilla, soft-serve (1/2 cup)	153	1	103	10	93	0.03

Granola bars

	VIT A (IU)	VIT C (mg)	CAL (mg)	MAG (mg)	PHOS (mg)	ZINC (mg)
Crunchy Almond/Brown Sugar, Low-fat, Kellogg (1 bar)	2381	0	35	87	248	2.2
Hard, chocolate chip (1 bar)	10	0	18	17	48	0.46
Hard, plain (1 bar, 1 oz.)	43	0	17	28	79	0.58
Nutri-Grain Cereal Bars, fruit, Kellogg (100 g)	2027	0	41	27	103	4.1
Soft, milk chocolate coating, chocolate chip (1 bar, 1.25 oz.)	14	0	37	23	70	0.46
Soft, milk chocolate coating, peanut butter (1 bar)	48	0	40	25	83	0.54
Soft, uncoated, nut and raisin (1 bar, 1 oz.)	12	0	24	26	68	0.45
Soft, uncoated, peanut butter (1 bar, 1 oz.)	4	0	26	24	71	0.53
Soft, uncoated, raisin (1 bar, 1.5 oz.)	0	0	43	31	94	0.55

Popcorn

	VIT A (IU)	VIT C (mg)	CAL (mg)	MAG (mg)	PHOS (mg)	ZINC (mg)
Air-popped (1 cup)	16	0	1	11	24	0.28
Air-popped, white popcorn (1 cup)	2	0	1	11	24	0.28

	VIT A (IU)	VIT C (mg)	CAL (mg)	MAG (mg)	PHOS (mg)	ZINC (mg)
Cakes (1 cake)	7	0	1	16	28	0.4
Caramel-coated, with peanuts (1 oz., ⅔ cup)	18	0	19	23	36	0.35
Caramel-coated, without peanuts (1 oz.)	14	0	12	10	24	0.16
Cheese-flavor (1 cup)	27	0	12	10	40	0.22
Oil-popped (1 cup)	17	0	1	12	28	0.29
White cheddar (1 cup)	114	2	28	21	*	*

Potato chips

	VIT A (IU)	VIT C (mg)	CAL (mg)	MAG (mg)	PHOS (mg)	ZINC (mg)
Made from dried potatoes, cheese flavor (1 oz.)	0	2	31	15	46	0.18
Made from dried potatoes, light (1 oz.)	0	3	10	18	44	0.17
Made from dried potatoes, plain (1 oz.)	0	2	7	16	45	0.17
Made from dried potatoes, sour cream and onion flavor (1 oz.)	214	3	18	16	48	0.2
Plain, light (1 oz.)	0	6	10	18	*	*
Plain, made with partially hydrogenated soybean oil, salted (1 cup)	0	71	54	152	375	2.47
Plain, unsalted (1 cup)	0	71	55	152	375	2.47
Potato sticks (1 oz.)	0	13	5	18	49	0.28

Pretzels

	VIT A (IU)	VIT C (mg)	CAL (mg)	MAG (mg)	PHOS (mg)	ZINC (mg)
Hard, plain, made with enriched flour, salted (1 oz.)	0	0	10	10	32	0.24

	VIT A (IU)	VIT C (mg)	CAL (mg)	MAG (mg)	PHOS (mg)	ZINC (mg)
Hard, plain, salted (1 oz.)	0	0	10	10	32	0.24
Hard, plain, salted (10 twists)	0	0	22	21	68	0.51
Hard, whole wheat (1 oz.)	0	0	8	9	35	0.18
Rice bar, crisped, chocolate chip (1 bar, 1 oz.)	500	0	6	14	38	0.24
Rice cakes, brown rice, multigrain, unsalted (1 cake)	0	0	2	12	33	0.23
Rice cakes, brown rice, plain (1 cake)	4	0	1	12	32	0.27
Rice Krispies Treats Squares, Kellogg's (100 g)	909	0	3	13	42	0.5

Snack bars (see also Granola bars)

	VIT A (IU)	VIT C (mg)	CAL (mg)	MAG (mg)	PHOS (mg)	ZINC (mg)
Chocolate (1 bar)	1166	21	29	19	*	*
Chocolate chip (1 bar)	1166	21	29	19	*	*
Chocolate chip crunch (1 bar)	500	9	150	24	*	*
Fat-free (1 bar)	333	*	20	*	*	*
Honey oats (1 bar)	833	*	0	24	*	8
Nutri-Grain (1 bar)	500	*	16	10	*	*
Peanut butter crunch (1 bar)	500	9	150	24	*	*
Vanilla crunch (1 bar)	500	9	150	24	*	*
Yogurt (1 bar)	67	9	60	*	*	*

SOUPS

	VIT A (IU)	VIT C (mg)	CAL (mg)	MAG (mg)	PHOS (mg)	ZINC (mg)
Bean with bacon (1 cup)	889	2	81	44	132	1.03
Beef bouillon, powder, dry (1 cube)	2	0	2	2	12	0
Beef broth, powder, dry (1 cube)	2	0	2	2	12	0
Beef noodle (1 cup)	629	0	15	6	46	1.54
Black bean canned, condensed, commercial (1 cup)	1144	1	90	85	193	2.83

	VIT A (IU)	VIT C (mg)	CAL (mg)	MAG (mg)	PHOS (mg)	ZINC (mg)
Black turtle soup, mature seeds, canned (1 cup)	10	7	84	84	259	1.3
Cheese, canned, condensed, commercial (1 cup)	2177	0	285	8	272	1.29
Chicken noodle, canned, condensed, commercial (1 cup)	1309	0	27	10	74	0.57
Chicken rice, canned, chunky, ready-to-serve (1 cup)	5858	4	34	10	72	0.96
Chicken Rice with Vegetables, canned, ready-to-serve, Progresso Healthy Classics (100 g)	688	0	10	10	37	0.18
Chicken vegetable, canned, chunky, ready-to-serve (1 cup)	5990	6	26	10	106	2.16
Chicken with dumplings, canned, condensed, commercial (1 cup)	1041	0	30	7	123	0.74
Chili beef, canned, condensed (1 cup)	3022	8	87	61	297	2.8
Clam chowder, Manhattan style, canned, chunky, ready-to-serve (1 cup)	3293	12	67	19	84	1.68
Clam chowder, New England, canned, condensed, commercial (1 cup)	20	5	82	15	85	1.51
Clam chowder, New England, made with milk (1 cup)	164	4	187	23	157	0.8
Consommé with gelatin, dehydrated, prepared (1 cup)	8	0	8	8	40	0
Corn chowder (1 cup)	450	39	73	31	*	*

	VIT A (IU)	VIT C (mg)	CAL (mg)	MAG (mg)	PHOS (mg)	ZINC (mg)
Crab, ready to serve (1 cup)	170	*	66	88	*	*
Cream of asparagus, canned, condensed, commercial (1 cup)	891	6	58	8	78	1.76
Cream of asparagus, canned, prepared with equal volume milk, commercial (1 cup)	600	4	174	20	154	0.93
Cream of broccoli, canned, ready-to-serve, Progresso Healthy Classics (100 g)	120	2	17	6	16	0.11
Cream of broccoli, Campbell's Restaurant Soup (½ cup)	0	12	80	*	*	*
Cream of celery, canned, condensed, commercial (1 cup)	612	1	80	13	75	0.3
Cream of celery, canned, prepared with equal volume milk, commercial (1 cup)	461	1	186	22	151	0.2
Cream of chicken, canned, condensed, commercial (1 cup)	1123	0	68	5	75	1.26
Cream of chicken, prepared with equal volume milk, commercial (1 cup)	714	1	181	17	151	0.68
Cream of mushroom, canned, condensed, commercial (1 cup)	0	2	65	10	85	1.19
Cream of mushroom, canned, prepared with equal volume milk, commercial (1 cup)	154	2	179	20	156	0.64

	VIT A (IU)	VIT C (mg)	CAL (mg)	MAG (mg)	PHOS (mg)	ZINC (mg)
Cream of potato, canned, condensed (1 cup)	577	0	40	3	93	1.26
Cream of potato, canned, prepared with equal volume milk, commercial (1 cup)	444	1	166	17	161	0.68
Cream of shrimp, canned, prepared with equal volume milk, commercial (1 cup)	313	1	164	22	146	0.8
Cream of vegetable, dehydrated, dry (1 packet)	27	3	24	9	40	0.28
Escarole, canned, ready-to-serve (1 cup)	2170	5	32	5	79	2.23
Gazpacho, canned, ready-to-serve (1 cup)	2604	7	24	7	37	0.24
Garlic and Pasta, canned, ready-to-serve, Progresso Healthy Classics (100 g)	1270	0	21	14	36	0.23
Lentil with ham, canned, ready-to-serve (1 cup)	360	4	42	22	184	0.74
Minestrone, canned, chunky, ready-to-serve (1 cup)	4351	5	60	14	110	1.44
Mushroom, dehydrated, dry (1 instant packet)	5	1	51	4	59	0.07
Mushroom, dehydrated, dry (1 regular packet)	22	4	228	18	263	0.3

	VIT A (IU)	VIT C (mg)	CAL (mg)	MAG (mg)	PHOS (mg)	ZINC (mg)
Onion mix, dehydrated, dry (1 packet)	8	1	55	25	126	0.23
Oyster stew, made with water	71	3	22	5	48	10.29
Oyster stew, made with milk (1 cup)	225	4	167	21	162	10.34
Pea, green, canned, prepared with equal volume milk, commercial (1 cup)	356	3	173	56	239	1.76
Pea, split, with ham, canned, chunky ready-to-serve (1 cup)	4872	7	34	38	178	3.12
Pepper pot (1 cup)	865	1	23	5	42	1.22
Tomato, canned, prepared with equal volume milk, commercial (1 cup)	848	68	159	22	149	0.29
Tomato and rice (1 cup)	755	0	23	5	33	0.51
Tomato beef with noodle (1 cup)	533	0	18	8	56	0.75
Tomato bisque, prepared with water (1 cup)	721	6	40	9	60	0.59
Tomato bisque, prepared with milk (1 cup)	879	7	186	25	174	0.63
Tomato bisque, with rice (1 cup)	755	15	23	5	33	0.51
Tomato bisque, with whole milk, (1 cup)	879	15	186	25	174	0.63
Tomato vegetable, prepared (1 cup)	850	5	8	20	*	*
Turkey noodle, canned, condensed commercial (1 cup)	585	0	23	10	95	1.17
Turkey, chunky (1 cup)	7156	6	50	*	104	2.12

	VIT A (IU)	VIT C (mg)	CAL (mg)	MAG (mg)	PHOS (mg)	ZINC (mg)
Vegetable with beef broth, canned condensed, commercial (1 cup)	4199	5	34	12	79	1.6
Vegetarian vegetable, canned, condensed, commercial (1 cup)	6034	3	42	15	69	0.92

SOY

	VIT A (IU)	VIT C (mg)	CAL (mg)	MAG (mg)	PHOS (mg)	ZINC (mg)
Fuyu, tofu, salted and fermented, prepared with calcium sulfate (1 block)	18	0	135	6	8	0.17
Koyadofu, tofu, dried-frozen (1 piece, 17 g)	88	0	62	10	82	0.83
Koyadofu, tofu, dried-frozen, prepared with calcium sulfate (1 piece, 17 g)	88	0	363	31	82	0.83
Miso, fermented soybeans (1 cup)	239	0	182	116	421	9.13
Natto, soybean product (1 cup)	0	23	380	201	305	5.3
Soybean, oil, salad or cooking (1 tbsp.)	0	0	0	0	0	0
Okara, tofu (1 cup)	0	0	98	32	73	0.68

Soybeans (see Soy for additional items)

	VIT A (IU)	VIT C (mg)	CAL (mg)	MAG (mg)	PHOS (mg)	ZINC (mg)
Boiled (½ cup)	8	6	88	74	211	0.99
Boiled (1 cup)	16	12	176	148	422	1.98
Dried, uncooked (½ cup)	22	6	257	261	654	4.54
Dried, uncooked (1 cup)	44	12	514	522	1308	9.08
Green, boiled, drained, without salt (1 cup)	281	31	261	108	284	1.64

	VIT A (IU)	VIT C (mg)	CAL (mg)	MAG (mg)	PHOS (mg)	ZINC (mg)
Green, fresh, boiled, drained (1/2 cup)	140	15	130	*	142	*
Green, fresh, raw (1/2 cup)	230	37	252	*	248	*
Green, raw (1 cup)	461	74	504	166	497	2.53
Mature seeds, boiled, with salt (1 cup)	16	3	175	148	421	1.98
Mature seeds, dry, roasted (1 cup)	40	8	464	392	1116	8.2
Mature seeds, roasted, salted (1 cup)	344	4	237	249	624	5.4
Mature seeds, sprouted, steamed (1 cup)	10	8	56	56	127	0.98
Mature seeds, sprouted, stir-fried (100 g)	17	12	82	96	216	2.1
Mature seeds, sprouted, raw (1/2 cup)	4	5	24	25	57	0.41
Organically produced, Arrowhead Mills, unprepared (1/4 cup)	0	0	100	*	*	*
Roasted (1/2 cup)	172	2	119	125	312	2.7
Soybean cakes						
Chinese style, extra firm (3 oz.)	0	0	150	*	*	*
Japanese style, firm (3 oz.)	0	0	150	*	*	*
Kinugoshi, silken (3 oz.)	0	0	20	*	*	*
Sprouted, raw (1/2 cup)	4	5	23	25	57	0.41
Sprouted, steamed (1/2 cup)	5	4	28	28	63	0.49

Soy Beverages

	VIT A (IU)	VIT C (mg)	CAL (mg)	MAG (mg)	PHOS (mg)	ZINC (mg)
Edensoy Organic Soy Beverage						
Carob, (1 cup)	*	*	68	43	105	0.64
Original (1 cup)	*	*	82	55	143	0.98
Original, Extra (1 cup)	1176	*	196	54	142	1
Vanilla (1 cup)	*	*	62	38	98	0.58

	VIT A (IU)	VIT C (mg)	CAL (mg)	MAG (mg)	PHOS (mg)	ZINC (mg)
Vanilla Extra (1 cup)	1176	*	196	38	294	0.57
Soy milk (1 cup)	77	*	10	45	117	0.54
Soy Moo, Fat-free, nondairy, lactose-free (1 cup)	0	0	400	*	*	*
Soy protein isolate (1 oz.)	0	0	50	11	220	1.14
Soy Protein Isolate Powder, Vitamin World, Isoflavones and Geristein, unprepared (1 scoop)	0	0	60	60	200	*
Tempeh (½ cup)	569	0	77	58	171	1.5
Tempeh, soybean product (1 cup)	1139	0	154	116	342	3.01
Tofu						
Fried, prepared with calcium sulfate (1 piece)	0	0	125	12	37	0.26
Koyadofu, dried-frozen (1 piece)	88	0	363	31	82	0.83
Koyadofu, dried-frozen (¼ lb)	587	1	412	67	545	5.5
Raw, firm (½ cup)	209	0	258	118	239	1.98
Raw, firm, prepared with calcium sulfate (½ cup)	209	0	861	73	239	1.98
Raw, regular (1 cup)	211	0	260	255	241	1.98
Raw, regular, prepared with calcium sulfate (½ cup)	105	0	434	37	120	0.99
Regular (½ cup)	105	0	130	127	120	1
Silken (3 oz.)	0	0	20	*	*	*
Silken, Lite, Low-Fat, Firm, Mori-Nu (3 oz.)	0	0	20	*	*	*

VEGETABLES, FRESH	VIT A (IU)	VIT C (mg)	CAL (mg)	MAG (mg)	PHOS (mg)	ZINC (mg)
Alfalfa seeds, fresh, sprouted (1 cup)	50	3	10	9	23	0.3
Artichoke, boiled (1 med.)	212	12	54	72	103	0.59
Artichoke hearts (½ cup)	149	8	38	51	72	0.44
Arugula, raw (½ cup)	237	2	16	5	5	0.06
Asparagus, boiled, drained (½ cup)	485	10	18	9	49	0.38
Balsam-pear, pods, boiled, drained (½ cup)	70	21	5	10	22	0.43
Balsam-pear, pods, boiled, drained (1 cup)	140	41	11	20	45	0.95
Bamboo shoots, boiled (½ cup)	0	0	7	2	12	*
Beans						
Adzuki, mature seeds, boiled (1 cup)	14	0	64	120	386	4.07
Baked, home-prepared (1 cup)	0	3	154	109	276	1.85
Black, mature seeds, boiled (1 cup)	10	0	46	120	241	1.93
Broad, immature seeds, boiled, drained (100 g)	270	20	18	31	73	0.47
Chickpeas (garbanzo beans bengal gram), mature seeds, boiled (1 cup)	44	2	80	79	276	2.51
Cranberry (Roman), mature seeds, boiled (1 cup)	0	0	89	89	239	2.02
French, mature seeds, boiled (1 cup)	5	2	112	99	181	1.13

	VIT A (IU)	VIT C (mg)	CAL (mg)	MAG (mg)	PHOS (mg)	ZINC (mg)
Great Northern, mature seeds, boiled (1 cup)	2	2	120	89	292	1.56
Kidney, California red, mature seeds, boiled (1 cup)	5	2	117	85	242	1.52
Kidney, all types, mature seeds, boiled (1 cup)	0	2	50	80	251	1.89
Limas						
Baby, frozen (1/2 cup)	150	5	25	50	101	0.5
Dried, boiled (1/2 cup)	0	0	16	41	104	0.89
Fresh (1/2 cup)	315	9	27	63	111	0.67
Fordhook, frozen (1/2 cup)	160	11	19	29	54	0.37
Mung, dehydrated (1 cup)	0	0	35	4	45	0.57
Mung, mature seeds, sprouted, raw (1 cup)	22	14	14	22	56	0.43
Navy, mature seeds, boiled (1 cup)	4	2	127	107	286	1.93
Pink, mature seeds, boiled (1 cup)	0	0	88	110	279	1.62
Pinto, immature seeds, frozen, boiled, drained (1/3 of 10 oz. package)	0	1	49	51	94	0.65
Pinto, mature seeds, boiled (1 cup)	3	4	82	94	274	1.85
Snap, green, boiled, drained (1 cup)	833	12	58	31	49	0.45
Snap, green, fresh, boiled (1/2 cup)	413	6	29	16	24	0.23
Snap, yellow, boiled (1 cup)	101	12	58	31	49	0.45

	VIT A (IU)	VIT C (mg)	CAL (mg)	MAG (mg)	PHOS (mg)	ZINC (mg)
Small white, mature seeds, cooked (1 cup)	0	0	131	122	303	1.95
Yam beans, fresh, raw, trimmed, sliced (1 cup)	25	24	14	14	21	0.19
Yard-long, fresh, boiled, drained, sliced (½ cup)	234	8	23	22	30	*
Yard-long, dried, boiled (½ cup)	14	*	36	84	156	0.92
Yellow, dried, boiled (½ cup)	2	2	66	61	152	0.98
White, regular, dried, boiled (½ cup)	0	0	81	57	102	1.24
White, small, boiled (½ cup)	0	0	66	61	152	0.98
Winged, boiled, drained (½ cup)	27	3	19	9	8	*
Winged, dried, boiled (½ cup)	0	0	122	47	132	1.24
Beet greens, raw (1 cup)	2318	11	45	27	15	0.14
Beets, boiled, drained (½ cup)	30	3	14	20	32	0.3
Bok choy, Chinese cabbage, cooked (1 cup)	5050	26	250	*	*	*
Broccoli						
Flowerets, raw (1 cup)	1095	66	34	18	47	0.28
Frozen, spears, boiled, drained (½ cup)	1741	37	47	18	51	0.28
Frozen, chopped, boiled, drained (1 cup)	3481	74	94	37	101	0.55
Brussels sprouts, frozen, boiled, drained (1 cup)	913	71	37	37	84	0.56

	VIT A (IU)	VIT C (mg)	CAL (mg)	MAG (mg)	PHOS (mg)	ZINC (mg)
Cabbage						
Boiled, drained (½ cup)	99	15	23	6	11	0.07
Chinese (pak-choi), boiled (1 cup)	4366	44	158	19	49	0.29
Chinese (pak-choi), raw (1 cup)	2100	32	74	13	26	0.13
Chinese (pe-tsai), boiled, drained, shredded (1 cup)	1151	19	38	12	46	0.21
Chinese (pe-tsai), raw, shredded (1 cup)	912	21	59	10	22	0.18
Marinated, Kim Chee (½ cup)	750	6	*	*	*	*
Raw (1 cup)	93	23	33	11	16	0.13
Red, boiled, drained, shredded (½ cup)	20	26	28	8	22	0.11
Red, raw, shredded (1 cup)	28	40	36	11	29	0.15
Savoy, raw, shredded (1 cup)	700	22	25	20	29	0.19
Swamp cabbage (skunk cabbage), raw, chopped (1 cup)	3528	31	43	40	22	0.1
Cactus, tender strips (2 tsp.)	100	*	*	*	*	*
Carrots						
Boiled, drained (½ cup, slices)	19,152	2	24	10	23	0.23
Raw (1 medium)	17,159	6	16	9	27	0.12
Raw, baby (1 medium)	197	1	2	1	4	0.02
Shredded (1 cup)	10,303	10	30	17	*	*
Cassava, raw (1 cup)	21	99	188	136	144	0.52
Cauliflower						
Frozen, boiled, drained (1 cup, 1″ pieces)	40	56	31	16	43	0.23

	VIT A (IU)	VIT C (mg)	CAL (mg)	MAG (mg)	PHOS (mg)	ZINC (mg)
Green, cooked (1/5 head)	127	65	29	17	51	0.57
Green, raw (1 cup)	97	56	21	13	40	0.41
Raw (1 cup)	19	46	22	15	44	0.28
Celeriac, raw (1 cup)	0	13	67	31	179	0.52
Celery, raw (1 cup, diced)	161	8	48	13	30	0.16
Chicory greens, raw, chopped (1 cup)	7200	43	180	54	85	0.76
Chicory roots, raw (1/2 cup, 1" pieces)	3	2	18	10	27	0.15
Chives, raw, chopped (1 tbsp.)	131	2	3	1	2	0.02
Collards, chopped, boiled, drained (100 g, or about 5/8 cup)	598	26	210	30	27	0.27
Corn						
Yellow, sweet, boiled, drained (1/2 cup cut)	178	5	2	26	84	0.39
Yellow, sweet, raw (1 medium ear)	253	6	2	33	80	0.41
White, frozen, kernels cut off cob, boiled (1/2 cup)	0	3	3	16	47	0.33
Cowpeas, common (black-eyed crowder, Southern), mature seeds, boiled (1 cup)	26	1	41	91	268	2.22
Cowpeas, cooked, chopped (1 cup)	305	10	37	33	22	0.13
Cress, garden, raw (1 cup)	4650	35	41	19	38	0.12
Cucumber, with peel, raw, slices (1/2 cup)	112	3	7	6	10	0.1
Dandelion greens, raw, chopped (1 cup)	7700	19	103	20	36	0.23

	VIT A (IU)	VIT C (mg)	CAL (mg)	MAG (mg)	PHOS (mg)	ZINC (mg)
Eggplant, boiled, drained, cubes (1 cup)	63	1	6	13	22	0.15
Endive, raw, chopped (½ cup)	513	2	13	4	7	0.2
Fennel, bulb, raw, sliced (1 cup)	117	10	43	15	44	0.17
Gingeroot, raw, sliced (¼ cup)	0	1	4	10	7	*
Horseradish, leafy tips, boiled, drained, chopped (1 cup)	2946	13	63	63	28	0.21
Horseradish-tree, pods, raw, slices (1 cup)	74	141	30	45	50	0.45
Hummus, garbanzo (½ cup)	31	10	62	36	138	1.35
Hummus, garbanzo (1 cup)	61	19	124	71	275	2.7
Jerusalem artichoke, raw, slices (1 cup)	30	6	21	26	117	0.18
Jicama, raw (1 cup)	25	43	17	13	32	*
Kale, boiled, drained, chopped (1 cup)	9620	53	94	23	36	0.31
Kale, frozen, boiled, drained, chopped (1 cup)	8260	33	179	23	36	0.23
Kohlrabi, boiled (1 cup)	29	44	20	16	39	*
Kohlrabi, raw (½ cup)	25	43	17	13	32	*
Leeks (bulb and lower leaf portion), drained, chopped, or diced, boiled (¼ cup)	12	1	8	4	4	0.02
Leeks (bulb and lower leaf portion), raw (1 cup)	85	11	53	25	31	0.11
Lentils, mature seeds, boiled (½ cup)	8	2	18	36	122	1.26
Lentils, mature seeds, boiled (1 cup)	16	3	38	71	356	2.52

	VIT A (IU)	VIT C (mg)	CAL (mg)	MAG (mg)	PHOS (mg)	ZINC (mg)
Lentils, sprouted, raw (1 cup)	35	13	19	29	133	1.16
Lettuce						
Butterhead (includes Boston and bibb types) raw, shredded (1 cup)	534	4	18	7	13	0.09
Cos, or romaine, raw, shredded (½ cup)	728	7	10	2	13	0.07
Iceberg, includes crisphead types, raw, shredded (1 cup)	182	2	11	5	11	0.12
Looseleaf, raw, shredded (½ cup)	532	5	19	3	7	0.08
Lotus root, raw (10 slices)	0	36	36	19	81	0.32
Mushroom						
Enoki, raw (1 large)	0	1	0	1	6	0.03
Raw, pieces or slices (1 cup)	0	3	4	7	73	0.51
Shiitake, dried (4 mushrooms)	0	1	2	20	44	1.15
White, raw, chopped (1 cup)	0	2	1	*	*	*
Mustard greens, boiled, drained, chopped (1 cup)	4243	35	104	21	57	0.15
Mustard greens, frozen, cooked, drained, chopped (1 cup)	6705	21	152	20	36	0.3
Mustard spinach, tendergreen, boiled, drained, chopped (1 cup)	14,760	117	284	13	32	0.2
Nopales, cooked (1 cup)	684	8	244	70	24	0.31
Okra, raw, sliced (1 cup)	660	*	81	57	63	0.6
Onions, dehydrated flakes (¼ cup)	0	11	36	13	42	0.27

	VIT A (IU)	VIT C (mg)	CAL (mg)	MAG (mg)	PHOS (mg)	ZINC (mg)
Onions, raw (1 large slice, ¼" thick)	0	2	8	3	13	0.07
Parsley, freeze-dried (¼ cup)	885	2	3	5	8	0.09
Parsley, raw (1 cup)	3120	80	82	30	35	0.64
Parsnips, raw, slices (1 cup)	0	23	48	39	94	0.79
Peas						
Cooked, podded (1 cup)	210	77	67	42	88	0.59
Green, boiled, drained (1 cup)	955	23	43	62	187	1.9
Green, frozen, boiled, drained (½ cup)	534	8	19	23	72	0.75
Split, dried, boiled (½ cup)	7	*	13	36	97	0.98
Split, mature seeds, boiled (1 cup)	14	1	27	71	194	1.96
Sprouted, mature seeds, raw (½ cup)	100	6	21	34	99	0.63
Peas and carrots, frozen, boiled, drained (½ cup)	6209	7	18	13	39	0.36
Peas and onions, frozen, boiled, drained (1 cup)	625	12	25	23	61	0.52
Peppers						
Hot chili, green, raw (1 pepper)	347	109	8	11	21	0.14
Hot chili, red, raw (1 pepper)	4838	109	8	11	21	0.14
Hot chili, sun-dried (1 pepper)	143	0	0	1	1	0.01
Sweet, red, raw (1 medium)	6783	226	11	12	23	0.14
Sweet, green, raw (1 medium)	752	106	11	12	23	0.14
Sweet, yellow, raw (1 large pepper)	443	341	21	22	45	0.32

	VIT A (IU)	VIT C (mg)	CAL (mg)	MAG (mg)	PHOS (mg)	ZINC (mg)
Pickle, cucumber, dill (1 large)	214	1	6	7	14	0.09
Pickle, cucumber, sweet (1 large)	44	0	1	1	4	0.03
Pigeon peas, mature seeds, cooked, boiled (1 cup)	5	0	72	77	200	1.51
Poi, taro root (1 cup)	16	10	37	58	*	*
Potatoes						
Boiled, cooked in skin, flesh (1 potato, 2½" dia.)	0	18	7	30	60	0.41
Boiled, cooked without skin (1 potato, 2½" dia.)	0	10	11	27	54	0.37
Raw, flesh and skin (1 large)	0	36	13	39	85	0.72
Pumpkin, boiled, drained, mashed (½ cup)	1320	6	18	11	37	*
Pumpkin, raw (1 cup, 1" cubes)	1856	10	24	14	51	0.37
Radicchio, raw, shredded (1 cup)	11	3	8	5	16	0.25
Radishes, raw, slices (½ cup)	5	13	12	5	10	0.17
Rhubarb, raw, diced (1 cup)	122	10	105	15	17	0.12
Rutabagas, raw, cubes (1 cup)	812	35	66	32	81	0.48
Seaweed						
Agar, dried (100 g)	0	0	625	770	52	5.8
Agar, raw (⅛ cup, 2 tbsp.)	0	0	5	7	1	0.06
Irishmoss, raw (⅛ cup, or 2 tbsp.)	12	0	7	14	16	0.2

	VIT A (IU)	VIT C (mg)	CAL (mg)	MAG (mg)	PHOS (mg)	ZINC (mg)
Kelp, raw (⅛ cup or 2 tbsp.)	12	0	17	12	4	0.12
Laver, raw (⅛ cup or 2 tbsp.)	520	4	7	0	6	0.11
Spirulina, dried (1 cup)	86	2	18	29	18	0.3
Spirulina, raw (1 cup)	56	1	12	19	11	0.2
Wakame, raw (⅛ cup or 2 tbsp.)	36	0	15	11	8	0.04
Shallots, fresh (1 tbsp.)	416	1	4	*	6	*
Spinach						
Cooked, drained (½ cup)	7471	9	124	74	51	0.68
Cooked, drained (1 cup)	14,742	18	245	157	101	1.37
Raw (1 cup)	2015	8	30	24	15	0.16
Frozen, chopped or leaf, boiled, drained (½ cup)	7395	12	139	66	46	0.67
Frozen, chopped or leaf, boiled, drained (1 cup)	7395	24	278	132	92	1.34
Squash						
Winter, acorn, baked, cubes (1 cup)	877	22	90	88	92	0.35
Winter, acorn, raw, cubes (½ cup)	238	9	23	23	25	0.09
Winter, acorn, raw, cubes (1 cup)	476	15	46	45	50	0.18
Winter, butternut, baked (½ cup)	7141	15	42	30	28	0.13
Winter, butternut, baked (1 cup)	14,282	31	84	60	55	0.26
Winter, butternut, frozen, boiled, mashed (½ cup)	4007	4	23	11	17	0.15
Winter, butternut, frozen, boiled, mashed (1 cup)	8014	8	46	22	34	0.3

	VIT A (IU)	VIT C (mg)	CAL (mg)	MAG (mg)	PHOS (mg)	ZINC (mg)
Winter, spaghetti, boiled or baked, drained, without salt (1/2 cup)	86	3	16	9	11	0.156
Winter, spaghetti, boiled or baked, drained, without salt (1 cup)	162	5	33	17	22	0.312
Zucchini						
Cooked (1/2 cup)	216	4	12	16	36	0.16
Cooked (1 cup)	432	8	24	38	72	0.32
Fresh, baby, raw (1 medium)	54	4	2	4	10	0.09
Frozen, boiled, drained, sliced (1/2 cup)	483	4	19	14	28	0.22
Frozen, boiled, drained, sliced (1 cup)	242	8	38	28	56	0.44
Succotash (corn and limas), boiled, drained (1 cup)	565	16	33	102	225	1.21
Sweet potatoes						
Baked in skin (1 large)	39,280	44	50	36	99	0.52
Boiled, without skin (1 medium)	25,752	26	32	15	41	0.41
Frozen, baked, cubes (1/2 cup)	24,441	8	31	14	34	0.27
Frozen, baked, cubes (1 cup)	28,882	16	62	37	77	0.53
Leaves, steamed, without salt (1/2 cup)	293	0	8	20	19	0.08
Leaves, steamed (1 cup)	586	1	15	39	38	0.17
Raw (1 potato, 5")	26,082	30	29	13	36	0.36
Swiss chard, boiled, drained, chopped (1 cup)	5493	32	102	151	58	0.58

	VIT A (IU)	VIT C (mg)	CAL (mg)	MAG (mg)	PHOS (mg)	ZINC (mg)
Taro, raw, sliced (1 cup)	0	5	45	34	87	0.24
Taro, Tahitian, raw, trimmed, sliced (½ cup)	1268	60	80	29	28	*
Taro leaves, steamed (½ cup)	3136	26	63	15	20	*
Taro shoots, raw, sliced (½ cup)	22	9	5	3	12	*
Tomatillo (1 medium)	39	4	4	13	25	0.15
Tomatillos, raw, chopped (½ cup)	75	8	5	13	26	0.15
Tomatoes						
Green, raw (1 medium)	790	29	16	12	34	0.09
Red, ripe, stewed (1 cup)	673	18	26	15	38	0.18
Red, ripe, raw, year-round average (1 medium whole, 1⅗″ dia.)	766	23	6	14	30	0.11
Sun-dried (1 cup)	472	21	59	105	192	1.08
Sun-dried (1 piece)	17	1	2	4	7	0.04
Sun-dried, oil-packed (1 cup)	1415	112	51	90	153	0.86
Sun-dried, oil-packed (1 piece)	39	3	1	2	4	0.02
Turnip, fresh, boiled, drained, mashed (½ cup)	0	13	26	9	22	*
Turnip greens, boiled, drained, chopped (1 cup)	7917	40	197	32	42	0.2
Turnip greens and turnips, frozen, boiled, drained (100 g)	5161	9	91	12	17	0.13
Water chestnuts, Chinese (matai), raw (½ cup)	0	3	7	14	39	0.31

	VIT A (IU)	VIT C (mg)	CAL (mg)	MAG (mg)	PHOS (mg)	ZINC (mg)
Watercress, raw, chopped (1 cup)	1598	15	41	7	20	0.04
Waxgourd, boiled, drained, cubed (½ cup)	0	18	32	*	30	*
Yams, boiled, drained (½ cup)	620	8	9	12	33	0.13
Yams, boiled, drained (1 cup)	1240	16	18	24	66	0.26
Yams, mountain, Hawaii, raw (½ cup, cubes)	*	1.77	17.9	8.2	23.1	0.16

VEGETABLES, CANNED

	VIT A (IU)	VIT C (mg)	CAL (mg)	MAG (mg)	PHOS (mg)	ZINC (mg)
Asparagus, drained solids (1 cup)	1285	45	39	24	104	0.97
Bamboo shoots, drained solids, slices (1 cup, ⅛″)	11	1	11	5	33	0.85
Beans						
Adzuki, mature seeds, sweetened (½ cup)	8	0	33	46	110	2.31
Adzuki, mature seeds, sweetened (1 cup)	15	0	65	92	219	4.62
Baked, plain or vegetarian (½ cup)	144	*	57	37	118	1.56
Baked, plain or vegetarian (1 cup)	388	*	114	73	236	3.17
Black, with liquid (½ cup)	5	3	42	42	130	0.65
Black, with liquid (1 cup)	10	6	84	84	269	1.3

	VIT A (IU)	VIT C (mg)	CAL (mg)	MAG (mg)	PHOS (mg)	ZINC (mg)
Broad (fava), mature seeds (½ cup)	13	3	34	41	101	0.8
Broad (fava), mature seeds (1 cup)	26	5	67	82	202	1.59
Chickpeas (garbanzos, bengal gram), mature seeds (½ cup)	29	5	39	35	108	1.27
Chickpeas (garbanzos, bengal gram), mature seeds (1 cup)	58	9	77	70	216	2.54
Cranberry (Roman), mature seed (½ cup)	0	1	44	42	112	1.09
Cranberry (Roman), mature seed (1 cup)	0	2	88	83	224	2.18
Great Northern, mature seeds (½ cup)	2	2	70	67	178	0.85
Great Northern, mature seeds (1 cup)	3	3	139	134	356	1.7
Hyacinth, cooked (½ cup)	44	5	20	18	22	*
Hyacinth, raw (1 cup)	88	10	40	36	44	*
Green, drained (½ cup)	300	4	18	9	13	0.2
Green, drained (1 cup)	599	7	36	18	26	0.4
Italian, green/yellow (½ cup)	80	2	18	9	*	*
Italian, green/yellow (1 cup)	159	4	35	18	*	*
Kidney, all types, mature seeds (½ cup)	0	2	35	40	135	0.7

	VIT A (IU)	VIT C (mg)	CAL (mg)	MAG (mg)	PHOS (mg)	ZINC (mg)
Kidney, all types, mature seeds (1 cup)	0	3	69	79	269	1.41
Kidney, red, mature seeds (½ cup)	0	2	31	36	121	0.7
Kidney, red, mature seeds (1 cup)	0	3	61	72	241	1.41
Lima, large, mature seeds (½ cup)	0	0	26	47	89	0.79
Lima, large, mature seeds (1 cup)	0	0	51	94	178	1.57
Mung, mature seeds sprouted, drained solids (½ cup)	15	0	9	6	20	0.18
Mung, mature seeds sprouted, drained solids (1 cup)	29	0	18	11	40	0.35
Navy, mature seeds (½ cup)	2	1	62	62	176	1.01
Navy, mature seeds (1 cup)	3	2	123	123	351	2.02
Pigeonpeas, boiled, drained (½ cup)	100	22	32	*	32	0.63
Pigeonpeas, boiled, drained (1 cup)	200	43	63	*	63	1.26
Pinto, mature seeds (½ cup)	2	1	52	33	111	0.83
Pinto, mature seeds (1 cup)	58	2	103	65	221	1.66
Refried, fat-free (½ cup)	0	8	45	42	108	1.47
Refried, fat-free (1 cup)	0	16	90	84	216	0.74
Refried, vegetarian (½ cup)	500	6	40	*	*	*
Refried, vegetarian (1 cup)	1000	12	80	*	*	*

	VIT A (IU)	VIT C (mg)	CAL (mg)	MAG (mg)	PHOS (mg)	ZINC (mg)
Shell, solids and liquids (½ cup)	280	4	36	19	37	0.33
Shell, solids and liquids (1 cup)	559	8	71	37	74	0.66
Snap, green, regular pack, drained solids (½ cup)	236	4	18	9	13	0.2
Snap, green, regular pack, drained solids (1 cup)	471	7	35	18	26	0.39
Snap, yellow, regular pack, drained, solids (½ cup)	71	3.5	18	9	13	0.2
Snap, yellow, regular pack, drained, solids (1 cup)	142	7	35	18	26	0.39
White, mature seeds (½ cup)	0	0	96	67	119	1.47
White, mature seeds (1 cup)	0	0	191	134	238	2.93
Bean sprouts (1 cup)	8	30	11	36	*	*
Beets						
Drained solids, slices (½ cup)	10	4	13	15	15	0.18
Drained solids, slices (1 cup)	19	7	26	29	29	0.36
Harvard, solids and liquids, slices (½ cup)	14	3	14	24	21	0.29
Harvard, solids and liquids, slices (1 cup)	27	6	27	47	42	0.57
Pickled, solids and liquids, slices (½ cup)	13	3	13	17	20	0.3
Pickled, solids and liquids, slices (1 cup)	25	5	25	34	39	0.59

	VIT A (IU)	VIT C (mg)	CAL (mg)	MAG (mg)	PHOS (mg)	ZINC (mg)
Carrots, regular pack, drained solids (½ cup)	10,055	2	19	6	18	0.19
Carrots, regular pack, drained solids (1 cup)	20,110	4	37	12	35	0.38
Corn						
Red and green peppers, solids and liquids (½ cup)	264	10	6	29	71	0.42
Red and green peppers, solids and liquids (1 cup)	527	20	11	57	141	0.84
White, sweet, cream-style, regular pack (½ cup)	0	6	4	22	66	0.68
White, sweet, cream-style, regular pack (1 cup)	0	12	8	44	131	1.36
Yellow, sweet, cream-style, regular pack (½ cup)	124	6	4	22	66	0.68
Yellow, sweet, cream-style, regular pack (1 cup)	248	12	8	44	131	1.36
Yellow, sweet, cream-style, special dietary pack (½ cup)	124	6	4	22	66	0.68
Yellow, sweet, cream-style, special dietary pack (1 cup)	248	12	8	44	131	1.36
Yellow, sweet, whole kernel, drained solids (½ cup)	128	7	4	17	54	0.32

	VIT A (IU)	VIT C (mg)	CAL (mg)	MAG (mg)	PHOS (mg)	ZINC (mg)
Yellow, sweet, whole kernel, drained solids (1 cup)	256	14	8	33	107	0.64
Cowpeas, common (black-eyed crowder, Southern), mature seeds plain (½ cup)	16	4	24	34	84	0.84
Cowpeas, common (black-eyed crowder, Southern), mature seeds plain (1 cup)	31	7	48	67	168	1.68
Hominy, white (½ cup)	0	0	8.5	23	29	0.87
Hominy, white (1 cup)	0	0	17	26	58	1.73
Hominy, yellow (½ cup)	88	0	8	23	28	0.84
Hominy, yellow (1 cup)	176	0	16	26	56	1.68
Hearts of palm (1 piece)	0	3	19	13	22	0.38
Mushrooms, drained solids (½ cup)	0	0	9	12	52	0.56
Mushrooms, drained solids (1 cup)	0	0	18	24	104	1.12
Olives, ripe (1 large)	18	0	4	0	0	0.01
Olives, ripe (10 large)	180	0	40	0	0	0.1
Peas, green, regular pack, drained solids (½ cup)	653	8	17	15	57	0.61
Peas, green, regular pack, drained solids (1 cup)	1306	16	34	29	114	1.21
Peas, seasoned, with liquid (½ cup)	494	13	18	17	61	0.74
Peas, seasoned, with liquid (1 cup)	988	26	36	34	122	1.48
Peas and carrots, regular pack, solids and liquids (½ cup)	7357	9	30	18	59	0.74
Peas and carrots, regular pack, solids and liquids (1 cup)	14,714	17	59	36	117	1.48

	VIT A (IU)	VIT C (mg)	CAL (mg)	MAG (mg)	PHOS (mg)	ZINC (mg)
Peas and onions, solid and liquids (½ cup)	97	2	10	10	31	0.04
Peas and onions, solid and liquids (1 cup)	193	4	20	19	61	0.7
Peppers						
Hot chili, green, pods, chopped, diced (½ cup)	415	46	5	10	12	0.12
Hot chili, green, pods, chopped, diced (1 cup)	830	92	10	20	24	0.24
Jalapeño, solids and liquids (½ cup chopped)	1156	9	18	8	12	0.13
Jalapeño, solids and liquids (1 cup chopped)	2312	18	35	16	23	0.26
Jute, potherb, raw (½ cup)	778	5	58	32	23	0.22
Jute, potherb, raw (1 cup)	1556	10	58	32	23	0.22
Sweet, green, solids and liquids, halves (½ cup)	109	33	29	8	24	0.13
Sweet, green, solids and liquids, halves (1 cup)	217	65	57	15	28	0.25
Pimento (1 whole)	1752	56	4	4	11	0.13
Potatoes, drained solids (½ cup)	0	5	5	13	35	0.25
Potatoes, drained solids (1 cup)	0	10	9	25	50	0.5
Pumpkin (½ cup)	26,908	5	32	28	42	0.21
Pumpkin (1 cup)	53,816	10	64	56	84	0.42
Pumpkin pie mix (½ cup)	11,202	5	50	22	61	0.37
Pumpkin pie mix (1 cup)	22,405	10	100	43	122	0.73
Sauerkraut, solids and liquids (½ cup)	13	11	22	10	24	0.14

	VIT A (IU)	VIT C (mg)	CAL (mg)	MAG (mg)	PHOS (mg)	ZINC (mg)
Sauerkraut, solids and liquids (1 cup)	26	21	43	19	28	0.27
Spinach, drained solids (½ cup)	9391	16	136	82	47	0.49
Spinach, drained solids (1 cup)	18,781	31	272	163	94	0.98
Spinach, New Zealand, raw (½ cup)	1232	8	16	11	9	0.11
Spinach, New Zealand, raw (1 cup)	2464	17	32	22	18	0.21
Squash, summer, crookneck, straightneck, drained solid, slices (½ cup)	131	3	13	14	23	0.32
Squash, summer, crookneck, straightneck, drained solid, slices (1 cup)	261	6	26	28	45	0.63
Squash, summer zucchini, Italian-style (½ cup)	612	3	20	16	33	0.30
Squash, summer zucchini, Italian-style (1 cup)	1224	5	39	32	66	0.59
Succotash (corn and limas) with cream-style corn (½ cup)	187.5	9	15	2	79	0.57
Succotash (corn and limas) with cream-style corn (1 cup)	375	17	29	3	157	1.14
Sweet potato, syrup pack, drained, solids (½ cup)	7014	11	17	12	25	0.15
Sweet potato, syrup pack, drained, solids (1 cup)	14,028	21	33	24	49	0.31
Sweet potato, vacuum pack, pieces (½ cup)	7988	27	22	22	49	0.18

	VIT A (IU)	VIT C (mg)	CAL (mg)	MAG (mg)	PHOS (mg)	ZINC (mg)
Sweet potato, vacuum pack, pieces (1 cup)	15,966	53	44	44	98	0.36
Tomato products						
Paste, without salt added (1 tbsp.)	4001	7	6	8	13	0.13
Puree, with salt added (1 cup)	3188	26	43	60	100	0.55
Red, ripe, stewed (1 cup)	1380	29	84	31	51	0.43
Red, ripe, wedges in tomato juice (1 cup)	1509	39	68	29	60	0.42
Red, ripe, with green chilies (1 cup)	940	15	48	27	34	0.31
Sauce, with mushrooms (1 cup)	2340	30	32	47	78	0.51
Sauce, with onions (1 cup)	2083	31	42	47	96	0.56
Sauce, with tomato tidbits (1 cup)	1954	53	24	49	103	0.46
Turnip greens, solids and liquids (½ cup)	4196	18	138	23	25	0.27
Turnip greens, solids and liquids (1 cup)	8292	36	276	46	50	0.54
Vegetables, mixed, drained solids (½ cup)	9493	4	22	13	35	0.34
Vegetables, mixed, drained solids (1 cup)	18,985	8	44	26	69	0.67
Water chestnuts, Chinese, solids and liquds (½ cup)	3	1	3	4	13	0.27
Water chestnuts, Chinese, solids and liquids (1 cup)	6	2	6	8	26	0.54

Section Three

SUPER BONE BOOSTERS— 102 RECIPES

APPETIZERS AND BEVERAGES

Appetizers

1. Date Nut Cherry Pâté
2. Fresh Basil and Tomato Salsa
3. Herbed Cheese Pita Chips
4. Hot and Spicy Chili Con Queso
5. Lime Yogurt Dip
6. Multivegetable Dip
7. Parmesan Spinach Dip
8. Red Potato Delight
9. Southwestern Bean and Cheese Dip
10. Spicy Black Bean Dip
11. Spicy Salmon Dip
12. Tomatoes and Mozzarella

Beverages

13. Fresh Orange Spritzer
14. Orange Julius Smoothie
15. Orange-Papaya Sunshine
16. Tomato-Lime Cooler
17. Yogurt Strawberry-Apricot Smoothie

BREADS AND MUFFINS

18. Cheddar Almond Muffins
19. French Camembert Bread
20. Fruited Scones
21. Heavenly Orange Ricotta Pancakes

22. Jalapeño Corn Bread
23. Spinach Bruschetta
24. Walnut Apricot Muffins

SALADS AND SAUCES

Salads

25. Americanized Greek Salad
26. Potato Salad
27. Carrot-Raisin Salad
28. Curried Rice and Chick Pea Salad
29. Feta Cabbage Salad
30. Four Greens and a Cheese Salad
31. Grilled Veggie Salad
32. Orange Fruit and Vanilla Cream
33. Orange Jicama Salad
34. Parmesan Sweet Basil and Bow Tie Salad
35. Spinach Gorgonzola Salad
36. Tabouli Salad
37. Waldorf Salad in Papaya Shell

Sauces

38. Béchamel Sauce (thick white sauce)
39. Fresh Basil and Creamy Parmesan Sauce
40. Tomato and Fresh Basil Sauce

MAIN DISHES

Beef

41. Beef and Chicken Medley
42. Beef Stroganoff
43. Southern Italian Meatballs

Poultry

44. Chicken Cacciatore
45. Chicken and Broccoli with Creamy Sun-Dried
    Tomato Sauce
46. Chicken and Yellow Rice
47. Curried Chicken and Fruit Salad

48. Mandarin Chicken
49. White Wine Chicken and Shrimp Newberg

Seafood

50. Ginger Salmon Florentine
51. Linguine and Salmon Italian
52. Mandarin Orange Shrimp in a Papaya
53. Shrimp and Vegetables in Sherry Cream
54. Smoked Salmon with Ginger Vinaigrette

SOUPS

55. Chilled Pineapple Gazpacho
56. Creamy Butternut Squash Soup
57. Healthy Vegetable Broth
58. Red, White, and Green Soup

PASTA AND RICE DISHES

59. Cheesy Chicken Manicotti
60. Confetti Brown Rice
61. Creamy Broccoli and Sun-Dried Tomatoes on Bow Ties
62. Four Vegetables and Cheese Risotto
63. Fresh Basil al Pomodoro Bow Ties
64. Gorgonzola Spinach with Couscous
65. Penne Pasta and Roasted Vegetables

VEGETABLES

66. Carrots and Sweet Potatoes
67. Julienne Vegetables with Lemon Butter
68. Lime Almond Brussels Sprouts
69. Mediterranean Garbanzos and Tomatoes
70. New Potatoes, Tomatoes, and Kale
71. One Potato, Two Potato, Three Potato, and More!
72. Orange Baked Squash
73. Spinach Cheddar Frittata

Soy

74. Broccoli, Potato, and Two Cheeses
75. Fruity Tofu Smoothie
76. Meatless Chili Crumble
77. Mexican Tempeh over Almond Rice
78. Soybeans
79. Soybean Bake
80. Three-Cheese Spinach and Tofu Lasagna
81. Sweet Tomato Cream
82. Wild Rice and Broccoli Cream

Desserts

83. Fresh Fruit Tartlet
84. Gourmet Fruit with Vanilla Bean Syrup
85. Guava Bread Pudding
86. Jewel's Apple Crumble
87. Layered Ambrosia
88. Light and Elegant Whipped Topping
89. Pumpkin Flan
90. White Chocolate Mousse

Quick and Easy Kids' Food

91. Crazy Kids' Mix
92. Orangeman Cupcakes

Picky Parties—A Bone-Boosting Party Snack
for Each Day of the Week

93. Picky Party 1—Sweet Treat
94. Picky Party 2—Nasty Nachos
95. Picky Party 3—Beans in a Bun
96. Picky Party 4—Veg-Out Bagel
97. Picky Party 5—Kiddie Quesadillas
98. Picky Party 6—Soft and Squeezy Tacos

Appetizers and Beverages

APPETIZERS

1. Date Nut Cherry Pâté

You need:

> 1 3-ounce package of fat-free or
>   light cream cheese
> 1 8-ounce container of marscapone
>   cheese
> ½ cup dates, chopped
> ¼ cup almonds, chopped (for pâté)
> 2 tablespoons maraschino cherries,
>   drained, chopped
> ¼ cup almonds, crushed (for
>   topping)
> Fresh fruit of choice (strawberries,
>   honeydew melon chunks, kiwi,
>   apple wedges, or papaya, among
>   many)
> A few sprigs of fresh mint

To make:

Let cream cheese soften while you prepare the pâté. In a medium-size bowl, cream marscapone cheese until soft. Gently stir in chopped dates, almonds, and cherries. In a separate bowl, mash cream cheese with a fork to soften. Mound cheese and fruit and nut mixture onto a round serving plate or tray, smoothing this into a rounded ball. Carve out the center of the mound, and spoon the cream cheese in the hole. Sprinkle the mound and cream cheese with crushed almonds, forming it into a more perfectly rounded shape. Use the fresh fruit of choice around the mound and sprigs of mint to decorate. Refrigerate until ready to serve, then let the pâté come to room temperature to soften. (You can wait to add the fresh fruit right before serving.) Makes 6 to 8 servings.

Doctor's ℞: Keep a food diary to see how many bone-boosting foods you eat each day. Can you see where your weaknesses lie? Determine how to add additional sources to your favorite meals, and make a plan to try one new bone-boosting recipe each day.

———————————

2. Fresh Basil and Tomato Salsa

You need:

> 2 large ripe tomatoes, finely chopped
> 6 green onions, chopped into ½-inch pieces
> 1 tablespoon fresh sweet basil
> 1 tablespoon fresh cilantro
> ½ teaspoon Salt Free Garlic and Herb Seasoning (McCormick)
> ½ teaspoon salt
> ½ teaspoon pepper
> 2 tablespoons jalapeño peppers, diced
> ½ cup pitted black olives, chopped
> 3 tablespoons fresh lime juice
> 1 tablespoon extra light olive oil

To make:

In a small bowl, combine tomatoes, green onions, spices, jalapeño peppers, black olives, lime juice, and extra light olive oil. Marinate covered for 1 hour in the refrigerator to combine flavors for best salsa taste. Serve with Herbed Cheese Pita Chips (next recipe). Makes 4 to 6 servings.

Chef's Comments: Add evaporated skim or nonfat milk to recipes that call for milk to double your calcium intake *without* doubling the fat calories.

———————

3. Herbed Cheese Pita Chips

You need:

- 4 large pita breads
- 2 tablespoons margarine
- 1 cup grated natural Parmesan cheese
- 1 teaspoon Salt Free Garlic and Herb Seasoning (McCormick)
- ¼ teaspoon onion powder
- ¼ teaspoon oregano

To make:

Preheat oven to 200 degrees. Separate pita bread by pulling apart to make eight rounds of bread; brush each side with margarine. Cut the rounds into fourths, then eighths. Combine Parmesan cheese and spices in a small bowl, then sprinkle over buttered pita. Place chips on a greased cookie sheet, and bake until crisp and golden. Cool completely and store airtight. Makes 64 chips.

4. Hot and Spicy Chili Con Queso

You need:

> 2 cups onions, finely chopped
> 1 tablespoon extra light olive oil
> 1 16-ounce can tomatoes, diced
> 1 4-ounce can green chilies,
>   chopped
> 1 4-ounce can tomato paste
> 1 tablespoon sugar
> 16 ounces low-fat cheddar cheese,
>   grated
> Salt and pepper to taste

To make:

In a medium sauce pan, sauté chopped onion over medium-high heat in the olive oil. Reduce temperature to medium low, and add tomatoes, chilies, tomato paste, sugar, cheese, and salt and pepper to taste. Continue stirring, and cook chili con queso for ½ hour on low to combine flavors. Serve with chips. Makes 8 to 10 servings.

5. Lime Yogurt Dip

You need:

> 4 ounces fat-free or light cream cheese,
>   softened
> 2 tablespoons confectioners sugar
> 1 8-ounce container vanilla yogurt
> 1 teaspoon lime zest (see page 278)
> ¼ teaspoon grated ginger (or
>   ginger powder)
> ½ teaspoon vanilla flavoring
> Assorted seasonal fruit to dip:
>   strawberries, apples, or melons

To make:

In a medium bowl, combine cream cheese and powdered sugar. Mix until creamy, slowly adding yogurt, vanilla, lime zest, and ginger. Beat until fluffy, and chill in refrigerator for 1 hour. Serve with assorted seasonal fruit. Cut slivers of lime peel for decoration, and lay this along the edge of the tray. Makes 6 to 8 servings.

Doctor's ℞: Researchers have found that those who eat soy protein instead of animal protein lose *50 percent less* calcium in the urine, thus helping to keep bones dense and strong. Because some Japanese women have half the rate of hip fractures as women in the United States, studies suggest that soy may be a key factor in helping to retain bone mass. How much soy is enough? Try to get at least one serving of soy each day (8 ounces of soy milk, ½ cup tofu, or ½ cup rehydrated textured vegetable protein).

6. Multivegetable Dip

You need:

> 1 8-ounce package fat-free or light
>   cream cheese
> ½ cup celery, chopped
> 4 green onions, diced
> 1 carrot, shredded
> ½ cup green bell pepper (or red or
>   yellow pepper), diced
> 1 8-ounce can water chestnuts,
>   chopped
> Dash onion powder
> Dash garlic powder
> Dash white pepper
> Vegetables of choice to dip

To make:

In a medium mixing bowl, combine cream cheese, celery, green onions, carrot, pepper, water chestnuts, and spices. Refrigerate for 1 to 2 hours to let flavors marinate, and serve with vegetables of your choice (celery, carrots, broccoli, cauliflower, bell peppers, and cherry tomatoes). Makes 8 servings.

Chef's Comments: Sprinkle sunflower seeds on vegetable casseroles to increase your magnesium intake, which is vital for bone health.

7. Parmesan Spinach Dip

You need:

> 3 tablespoons onion, chopped
> 1 tablespoon extra light olive oil
> 2 tablespoons flour
> ½ cup fat-free or low-fat calcium-
> fortified milk
> ½ cup fat-free or light sour cream
> 2 10-ounce packages frozen
> spinach, cooked, drained
> 6 ounces natural Parmesan cheese,
> grated
> ½ teaspoon pepper
> ½ teaspoon garlic powder
> ½ teaspoon celery seed
> 1 tablespoon Worcestershire sauce

To make:

In a medium sauce pan, sauté onion in olive oil on medium-high heat until soft. Add flour, followed by milk and sour cream, stirring until thickened. Reduce temperature to medium. Stir in spinach, cheese, spices, and Worcestershire sauce, stirring until cheese is melted. Serve hot with corn chips, or you can chill the dip and serve with fresh crudités. Makes 8 servings.

8. Red Potato Delight

You need:

>   2 pounds red potatoes
>   ½ teaspoon Aunt Jane's Crazy Salt
>   (or Mrs. Dash)
>   8 ounces fat-free or low-fat sour
>   cream
>   1 teaspoon Salt Free Garlic and
>   Herbs Seasoning (McCormick)
>   ½ teaspoon onion powder
>   ½ teaspoon garlic powder
>   Pepper, to taste
>   1 cup low-fat sharp cheddar cheese
>   (or cheese of your choice),
>   grated
>   1 tablespoon fresh chives

To make:

In a medium-size pot, cover potatoes with water. Add ½ teaspoon Aunt Jane's Crazy Salt, and boil over medium-high heat until soft (about 12 minutes). Drain, and run cool water over potatoes. In a small mixing bowl, whip sour cream, Salt Free Garlic and Herb Seasoning, onion powder, garlic powder, and pepper; set aside. Scoop out the center of the cooled potatoes, making a "well," then fill each with the sour cream mixture; top with grated cheese. Broil the potatoes just before serving to melt cheese, then serve on a platter with fresh herbs such as chives for garnish. These make great finger foods for children and teens. Makes 6 to 8 servings.

Variations:

- Garnish with fresh basil, oregano, or cilantro.
- Substitute 1 cup plain yogurt for the sour cream.
- Drain and flake one 8-ounce can of salmon and add to sour cream filling, reducing sour cream to ¾ cup.

9. Southwestern Bean and Cheese Dip

You need:

> 8 ounces fat-free or low-fat cream cheese
> 8 ounces silken tofu
> 1 teaspoon cumin
> 8 ounces fat-free or low-fat sour cream
> 16 ounces fat-free vegetarian refried beans
> 1 cup chopped green onions
> ½ cup pitted black olives, sliced
> 1 cup low-fat cheddar cheese, grated
> 2 tomatoes, chopped

To make:

Beat cream cheese, tofu, and cumin until blended. Spread in bottom of a 9×13-inch pan. Spread sour cream on top of this, then cover with a thin layer of refried vegetarian beans. Sprinkle with chopped green onions, sliced olives, grated cheese, and chopped tomatoes. Serve with low-fat baked tortilla chips or chopped vegetables. Makes 8 to 12 servings.

Variations:

- Add ¾ pound browned then drained ground round or ground turkey on top of refried vegetarian beans.
- Substitute fat-free or low-fat calcium-fortified cottage cheese for the cream cheese. Process until smooth; add tofu and cumin, and process again.
- Add your favorite salsa between layers.
- Spoon 10 ounces cooked and drained spinach between layers
- Buy tofu prepared with calcium sulfate, since it delivers more bone-boosting calcium.
- Use 10 to 12 chopped sun-dried tomatoes for a power punch of vitamin C.

10. Spicy Black Bean Dip

You need:

> 1 15-ounce can black beans, rinsed,
>   drained
> ½ cup green onions, chopped
> 1 cup Fresh Basil and Tomato
>   Salsa (page 166)
> 1 teaspoon chili powder
> ½ teaspoon cumin
> ¼ cup fresh cilantro
> 1 tablespoon lime juice
> ½ cup low-fat sharp cheddar
>   cheese, grated

To make:

In a medium bowl, combine rinsed and drained black beans, green onions, Fresh Basil and Tomato Salsa, chili powder, cumin, cilantro, and lime juice. Pour into a medium saucepan, and cook for 7 minutes on medium heat. Pour into a serving bowl; top with grated cheddar cheese. Serve immediately with Herbed Cheese Pita Chips (page 167). Makes 8 servings.

Doctor's ℞: Along with eating a diet high in bone-boosting nutrients, be sure to engage in weight-bearing exercise such as walking, jumping rope, aerobics, stair climbing or jogging. This will let you lose unwanted fat while also building bone strength.

———————

11. Spicy Salmon Dip

You need:

> 1 8-ounce package of fat-free or
>   light cream cheese (softened)
> 1 8-ounce can salmon, drained
> ½ cup fat-free or light sour cream
> ½ teaspoon hot sauce
> ¼ cup green onions, chopped
> ½ teaspoon white pepper
> ½ teaspoon Salt Free Garlic and
>   Herb Seasoning (McCormick)
> 1 tablespoon horseradish

To make:

In a small serving bowl combine cream cheese, drained and flaked salmon, sour cream, hot sauce, green onions, pepper, Salt Free Garlic and Herb Seasoning, and horseradish. Serve with pumpernickel or whole wheat cocktail bread slices, veggies, Herbed Cheese Pita Chips, or your favorite chip. Make 6 to 8 servings.

Variations:

- Substitute calcium-fortified, low-fat cottage cheese for the cream cheese. Blend in a food processor until smooth, then add to the recipe.
- Eliminate horseradish, and add favorite herbs such as basil or cilantro.
- Add 1 chopped tomato, or try 10 chopped sun-dried tomatoes.
- Use 8 ounces silken tofu instead of sour cream for extra bone-boosting benefits.

Chef's Comments: A mango has nearly 10,000 IUs of vitamin A, as well as being rich in zinc and magnesium. Slice these super bone boosters, and add to meals for extra nutrients.

12. Tomatoes and Mozzarella

You need:

>4 tablespoons olive oil
>2 tablespoons balsamic vinegar
>1 teaspoon garlic powder
>1 teaspoon onion powder
>Salt and pepper to taste
>⅛ cup basil, fresh
>⅛ cup oregano, fresh
>3 large tomatoes, cut into ¼″ slices
>8 ounces mozzarella cheese, partial
>   skim, cut in ¼″ slices

To make:

Cover the bottom of a serving tray or platter with 2 table-spoons olive oil, 1 tablespoon balsamic vinegar, ½ teaspoon garlic powder, and ½ teaspoon onion powder. Add a dash of salt and pepper, then mix together. Sprinkle all but 2 tablespoons chopped fresh basil and oregano on top of this. Put sliced tomatoes in a single layer; top with cheese slices. Lightly sprinkle tomatoes and cheese with salt, pepper, ½ teaspoon garlic powder, and ½ teaspoon onion powder. Sprinkle with 2 tablespoons olive oil and 1 tablespoon balsamic vinegar, then dot with the remaining oregano and basil. Cover with plastic wrap, and marinate in the refrigerator up to four hours. For best flavor, allow salad to set at room temperature for 1 hour before serving. Makes 8 servings.

Variations:

- Substitute Parmesan, Monterey Jack, feta, or Colby for the mozzarella cheese.
- Add a layer of thinly sliced cucumbers over tomatoes.
- Add a layer of thinly sliced sweet onion over tomatoes, then add cheese slices.

BEVERAGES

13. Fresh Orange Spritzer

You need:

> 4 ounces fresh orange juice,
>   strained
> 1 tablespoon fresh lemon juice,
>   strained
> 8 ounces seltzer water, chilled
> 1 maraschino cherry (for garnish)
> 1 thin orange slice (for garnish)

To make:

Pour first three ingredients in a large glass and stir. Add ice cubes, and top with cherry and orange slice. Makes 1 serving.

Variations:

- Use citrus ice cubes (1 part orange, lemon, or lime juice to 3 parts water; combine, and freeze into cubes).

14. Orange Julius Smoothie

You need:

> 8 ounces calcium-fortified orange
>   juice
> 4 ounces frozen orange juice
>   concentrate
> 3 tablespoons sugar
> 1 frozen banana, cut in chunks
> 1 teaspoon vanilla extract
> 3 frozen milk cubes (see page 289)

To make:

Place all ingredients in a blender or food processor, and blend until creamy. If you prefer a thicker drink, add more frozen milk cubes. Makes 2 servings.

Variations:

- Substitute soy milk for skim milk when making frozen cubes, or use ½ soy milk, ½ skim milk.
- Use ½ cup nonfat plain or fruited yogurt to replace ½ cup of the calcium-fortified orange juice.
- Substitute 1 cup pineapple chunks for banana.

15. Orange-Papaya Sunshine

You need:

> 1 8-ounce container fat-free or low-fat vanilla yogurt
> ½ cup orange juice
> ½ papaya, peeled and chopped
> 4 ice cubes prepared with soy milk or skim milk (see page 289)
> Honey or sugar to sweeten to taste

To make:

Place all ingredients in a blender or food processor, and blend until creamy. If you prefer a thicker drink, add more frozen milk cubes. Makes 2 servings.

Variations:

- Add a banana to thicken and sweeten the shake.
- Substitute 8 ounces of silken tofu for the yogurt. Sweeten to taste.

Doctor's ℞: Increase your intake of magnesium by including black beans, chickpeas, kidney beans, and broad beans in your daily diet. Or sprinkle sunflower seeds on your baked potato or favorite salad.

———————

16. Tomato-Lime Cooler

You need:

> 8 ounces low-sodium tomato juice
> ½ lime, squeezed into blender
> 4 lime juice ice cubes (1 part lime
>   juice to 3 parts water; combine,
>   and freeze into cubes)

To make:

Place all ingredients in a blender or food processor; blend and serve. Makes 1 serving.

Chef's Comments: Fill sandwiches with romaine lettuce. Just ½ cup of romaine gives you 728 IUs of vitamin A.

17. Yogurt Strawberry-Apricot Smoothie

You need:

> 1 8-ounce container vanilla fat-free
> or low-fat yogurt
> ½ cup frozen strawberries
> 2 fresh apricots (discard pits)
> ½ cup fat-free or low-fat calcium-
> fortified milk (or soy milk)

To make:

Put all ingredients in a blender or food processor, and blend until creamy. If you prefer a thinner drink, add frozen milk cubes (page 289) or citrus cubes (page 177). Makes 2 servings.

Variation:

- Substitute 8 ounces of silken tofu for the yogurt. Sweeten to taste.

Breads and Muffins

18. Cheddar Almond Muffins

You need:

> 2 cups all-purpose flour
> 1 tablespoon sugar
> 1 tablespoon baking powder
> ½ teaspoon nutmeg
> ½ teaspoon salt
> 1¼ cups fat-free or low-fat calcium fortified milk
> ¼ cup vegetable oil
> 2 ounces egg substitute (or 1 large egg)
> 4 ounces low-fat sharp cheddar cheese, grated
> ½ cup sliced almonds
> ½ apple, with peel, chopped

To make:

Preheat oven to 400 degrees; grease a muffin tin, or use muffin papers. In a large bowl, combine flour, sugar, baking powder, nutmeg, and salt. In a small bowl, combine milk, oil, and egg substitute until blended. Add milk mixture to dry ingredients, stirring until moistened. Fold in all but 2 tablespoons of the cheese (reserve for topping), almonds, and chopped apple. Spoon mixture into muffin cups. Bake in the center of the oven for 15 to 20 minutes, or until light brown. Sprinkle 2 tablespoons of cheese over muffins while they are hot. Cool slightly and serve warm. Makes 12 muffins.

Variations:

- Serve muffins with warm orange or honey butter.

19. French Camembert Bread

You need:

> 1 loaf French bread (buy fresh
> from the bakery)
> ½ stick reduced-calorie margarine
> (or regular margarine or butter)
> 4 ounces Camembert cheese
> 3 tablespoons fresh parsley
> Dash garlic powder
> Salt and pepper to taste

To make:

Preheat oven to 400 degrees. Cut bread in ¾-inch slices without cutting completely through the bread. In a medium bowl, cream the butter and cheese. Add the parsley and garlic, and season with salt and pepper to taste. Spread the cheese mixture on each side of each slice of bread. Wrap in foil; bake for 20 minutes for soft bread. For crisper bread, open the foil the last few minutes of baking time. Makes one loaf.

20. Fruited Scones

You need:

> 2 cups whole wheat flour
> ¼ teaspoon salt
> 6 tablespoons margarine
> ¾ cup sugar
> ½ cup chopped dried fruit such as
>   raisins, golden currants, apricots,
>   peaches, apples, dried blueberries,
>   cherries, or cranberries
> ½ cup fat-free or low-fat calcium-
>   fortified milk
> Optional: ¼ cup slivered almonds,
>   pecans, or walnuts, chopped

To make:

Preheat oven to 425 degrees. In a large bowl, combine flour and salt. Cut softened margarine into the flour mixture until crumbly. Stir in the sugar and fruit (nuts are optional). Add milk, and stir gently until moist. Roll dough out about ¾-inch thick and cut into 3-inch rounds, using a biscuit cutter or glass with a 3-inch diameter. (Dust the glass rim in flour each time before cutting scone, and it will not stick to the dough.) Place rounds close together on a lightly greased baking sheet, and bake for 10 to 15 minutes or until golden brown. Cool on a wired rack and serve warm. Makes 12 scones.

Variations:

- Add 1 teaspoon orange zest (page 278).
- Try ¼ cup oil-packed sun-dried tomatoes, drained and chopped, instead of fruit.
- Combine 1 teaspoon cinnamon with 1 tablespoon sugar. Sprinkle this on top before cooking.

Doctor's ℞: What do you choose for a midafternoon snack? One cup of plain yogurt contains 450 milligrams of calcium—almost 50 percent of your daily requirement—and six dried figs contain 160 milligrams of calcium. Remember this when you are thinking about eating that candy bar or package of chips, and do your bones a favor!

———————————

21. Heavenly Orange Ricotta Pancakes

You need:

> 2 oranges
> ¾ cup fat-free or low-fat plain yogurt
> ½ cup fat-free or low-fat ricotta cheese
> 4 ounces egg substitute (or 2 large eggs)
> ¾ cup all-purpose flour
> ½ teaspoon baking soda
> ¼ teaspoon salt
> ½ teaspoon orange zest (page 278)
> Cooking spray
> ¼ cup sifted powdered sugar

To make:

Peel oranges, and pull apart into segments. Arrange 4 to 5 segments along one side of each individual plate (domino style); set aside, and prepare pancakes. In a blender or food processor, combine yogurt, ricotta, and egg substitute. Blend completely until smooth. Stir flour, baking soda, salt, and orange zest; add to yogurt mixture. Process again until blended. Spray pancake griddle or skillet with cooking spray, and heat to medium-high. Add pancake mixture quickly before cooking spray starts to smoke, cooking several pancakes at a time. When bubbles appear on the top of the pancake, turn, and brown the other side. Put two to three pancakes on each plate next to orange segments. Sprinkle entire plate, oranges, and pancakes with powdered sugar for a beautiful presentation. Makes 8 to 10 pancakes.

Variations:

- Substitute soy flour for part of the all-purpose flour.

Chef's Comments: Choose light mayonnaise for favorite sandwiches and salad dressings. One tablespoon has 25 percent of your daily requirement of vitamin K.

22. Jalapeño Corn Bread

You need:

2½ cups yellow cornmeal
1 cup regular enriched flour
2 tablespoons sugar
4 teaspoons baking powder
½ teaspoon salt
1½ cups fat-free or low-fat
  calcium-fortified milk
6 ounces egg substitute (or 3 large
  eggs)
½ cup extra light olive oil
1 15-ounce can creamed corn
6 to 8 chilies, chopped
1¼ cups low-fat sharp cheddar
  cheese, cubed
1 large onion, chopped

To make:

Preheat oven to 425 degrees. Mix cornmeal, flour, sugar, baking powder, and salt in a large bowl. Add milk, egg substitute (or beaten eggs), olive oil, creamed corn, chopped chillies, cubed cheese, and chopped onion. Stir all ingredients, then pour into two well-greased 9×13-inch pans. Bake for 25 minutes, or until done in the center. Makes 24 squares. Freezes well.

Variations:

- Substitute Monterey Jack, Colby, or Parmesan cheese for the sharp cheddar cheese.
- For a milder cornbread, eliminate the chopped chilies.
- Sprinkle additional grated cheese on top of cornbread during last five minutes of baking.
- Consider soy flour for ¼ cup of the all-purpose flour. Cooking time may vary as soy flour browns more quickly.

23. Spinach Bruschetta

You need:

> 1 garlic clove
> 2 cups fresh spinach or 1 10 oz.
>   package of frozen spinach
> 3 tablespoons extra light olive oil
> Salt and pepper to taste
> 2 large tomatoes, finely chopped
> 1 red onion, small, finely chopped
> ½ loaf French bread
> ½ cup Parmesan cheese, grated
> ¼ cup basil, fresh
> ¼ cup oregano, fresh

To make:

In a small bowl, crush garlic with a fork; pour in olive oil. Allow this to marinate while you prepare the bread topping. Cook fresh or frozen spinach in a medium-size pot with ¼ cup water, and drain. Salt and pepper spinach to taste, then blot with a paper towel to ensure that it is liquid-free. Combine spinach with chopped tomatoes and onions; drain liquid, and add 1 tablespoon olive oil marinade. Slice bread ½″ thick; place pieces on a lightly greased cookie sheet. Brush bread lightly with remaining olive oil marinade, and broil for 1 minute until slightly crisp. Remove bread from oven. In the center of each piece of bread, put 1 tablespoon of the spinach mixture, topped with a sprinkle of Parmesan cheese, basil, and oregano. Top this with another tablespoon of the spinach mixture; sprinkle lightly with remaining cheese, basil, and oregano. Broil for 1 to 2 minutes until bubbly but not too brown; serve hot. Makes 6 to 8 servings.

Variations:

- Use chopped sun-dried tomatoes in addition to tomatoes, or as a substitution.

- Add chopped mushrooms to tomato and onion mixture.
- Substitute reduced-fat cheese such as mozzarella, feta, or Romano.

24. Walnut Apricot Muffins

You need:

> 2 cups all-purpose flour
> ½ cup sugar
> 1 tablespoon baking powder
> ½ teaspoon salt
> 1 teaspoon orange zest (page 278)
> ½ cup dried apricots, chopped
> ½ cup walnuts, chopped
> ½ cup fat-free or low-fat sour cream
> ½ cup fat-free or low-fat calcium-fortified milk
> ½ cup margarine, melted
> 2 ounces egg substitute (or 1 egg, beaten)

Icing

> 1 to 2 medium oranges (make 2 tablespoons of orange zest, then juice oranges)
> 1 lemon (make 1 tablespoon lemon zest, then juice lemons)
> 1 16-ounce box confectioners' sugar

To make:

Preheat oven to 400 degrees. Grease muffin cups, or use muffin papers. Clean oranges and lemon, and make zest. Put zest aside, and continue with recipe. In a large bowl, combine flour, sugar, baking powder, salt, 1 teaspoon orange zest (hold remaining lemon and orange zest for icing), apricots, and walnuts. In a small bowl, combine sour cream, milk, margarine, and egg substitute. Stir the sour cream mixture into the flour mixture until moistened, then spoon into prepared greased muffin tin cups. Bake on the center rack of the oven for 15 to 20 minutes (medium-sized muffins). While the muffins are cooking, make the icing, combining confectioners' sugar, zest, and ½ cup of combined lemon and orange juices. Blend together, and hold until muffins are done. Using a knife, stick the tip into the center of one muffin to make sure it is thoroughly cooked. The knife should come out clean, and the top of the muffin should be golden. Cool muffins for several minutes, then using a glove, carefully lift out muffins, dipping each top into the icing. Arrange on a plate, and serve warm. Wrap remaining muffins in foil, and freeze for future use. Makes 12 muffins.

Salads and Sauces

25. Americanized Greek Salad

You need:

- 4 cups romaine lettuce, cleaned, patted dry
- ½ cup green onions, chopped
- 2 medium tomatoes, sliced into bite-size pieces
- ½ cup black olives, sliced
- 1 cucumber, cut into 2-inch sticks about ½-inch thick, with or without peel
- 2 celery stalks, cut in 2 inch strips
- 8 baby carrots
- 4 radishes, decoratively cut across the top like a tic-tac-toe board
- ½ cup pickled beets
- 2 tablespoons fresh basil
- 4 ounces feta cheese

26. Potato Salad

You need:

- 8 medium potatoes, peeled, chopped into bite-size pieces
- ½ teaspoon salt in cooking water
- ½ cup fat-free or low-fat mayonnaise
- ¼ cup fat-free or light sour cream
- ½ teaspoon salt
- ½ teaspoon pepper
- Dash garlic powder

Dressing

> ¼ cup extra light olive oil
> ½ cup white wine vinegar

To make salads:

Put peeled and chopped potatoes in a medium pot. Cover with water and ½ teaspoon salt. Boil on medium-high heat for 12 minutes. Potatoes are done when the large pieces are soft in the middle. Pour into a colander to drain potatoes, and cool under water. Drain again. Put potatoes into a medium bowl and stir in mayonnaise, sour cream, salt, pepper, and garlic. Refrigerate while you prepare the vegetables. (You can make the potato salad the day before, then prepare the green salad right before serving.) Cut vegetables, according to the directions given on page 192. On a large decorative serving tray (approximately 15 inches or larger), layer half of the lettuce, covering the whole tray. Mound the potato salad into the center of the tray. Cover potato salad with the remaining lettuce. Decorate with the prepared vegetables. For example, place green onions around the top of the potato salad, tomatoes around the base of the potato salad, and black olives over the tomatoes. Use the cucumber sticks, celery sticks, and baby carrots to spread around the potato salad, then layer the beets decoratively on top. Sprinkle fresh basil over entire dish, and then add the crumbled feta. To make the dressing: In a small bowl, combine olive oil and vinegar. Pour one-half of this over the entire salad. Serve the other half of the dressing, if needed, for individual servings. Makes 8 servings.

Doctor's ℞: People who eat calcium-rich foods are less likely to develop kidney stones than those who consume smaller amounts of these foods. However, those who take calcium supplements are more likely to develop kidney stones than those who do not take supplements. More reason to eat bone-boosting foods!

———————

27. Carrot-Raisin Salad

You need:

>   8 medium carrots (grate in
>   processor or by hand)
>   1 8-ounce can crushed pineapple
>   (drained)
>   ½ cup golden raisins
>   1 golden delicious apple (chopped
>   with peel)
>   ⅓ cup fat-free or low-fat
>   mayonnaise
>   2 tablespoons lemon juice
>   ½ cup walnut pieces

Variations:

• Substitute chopped peanuts or almonds for walnuts.

To make:

In a medium-size bowl, combine carrots, crushed pineapple, raisins, apple, mayonnaise, and lemon juice. Toss all ingredients (except walnuts); cover, and refrigerate for 1 hour. Add chopped walnuts, and serve. Makes 4 servings.

Chef's Comments: Sweets can have some bone-boosting benefit. Did you know that one cup of brown sugar has 187 milligrams of calcium?

28. Curried Rice and Chickpea Salad

You need:

> 2 cups brown rice, prepared according to package directions
> 1 15-ounce can chickpeas, rinsed, drained
> 1 bell pepper (green, red, or yellow), finely chopped
> ½ cup golden currants
> 2 carrots, grated
> ½ cup walnuts, chopped
> 2 tablespoons green onions, chopped
> 1 tablespoon fresh cilantro or chives (optional)

Dressing

> ¾ cup fat-free or light sour cream
> 2 tablespoons fat-free or low-fat mayonnaise
> 1 tablespoon lemon juice
> 1 teaspoon curry powder
> Dash garlic powder
> Salt and pepper to taste

To make:

In a medium saucepan, prepare brown rice according to package directions, adding chickpeas before covering. When the chickpeas and rice are ready, pour into a medium bowl. Combine bell pepper, currants, carrots, walnuts, and green onions, and add to chickpeas and rice. Add cilantro or chives. To make dressing: In a small bowl combine sour cream, mayonnaise, lemon juice, curry, and garlic; salt and pepper to taste. Pour over rice and vegetables, stir thoroughly, and serve. Makes 4 to 6 servings.

Variations:

- Substitute ¼ cup of silken tofu for ¼ cup sour cream. Mix in a blender with dressing ingredients until smooth.

29. Feta Cabbage Salad

You need:

>   1 head green cabbage
>   1 medium red onion
>   2 cucumbers
>   1 can large pitted black olives
>   8 to 10 sun-dried tomatoes
>   6 ounces feta cheese
>   ½ teaspoon salt
>   ½ teaspoon pepper
>   2 tablespoons fresh basil (or dried)
>   Extra light olive oil (to taste)
>   Vinegar (to taste)

To make:

Using your food processor or cutting board, chop cabbage, red onion, and cucumbers into bite-size pieces and mix together in a large bowl. Slice olives; add to chopped vegetables, then add sun-dried tomatoes. Crumble feta cheese on top. Add salt, pepper, and basil. Toss ingredients with oil and vinegar to taste. Will keep in refrigerator for 24 hours. Serves 10 to 12.

Variations:

- Add other fresh vegetables such as green pepper, chopped fresh spinach, or radishes.
- Use favorite herbs such as cilantro or chives to give added flavor.

30. Four Greens and a Cheese Salad

You need:

> 1 cup romaine lettuce
> 1 cup arugula
> 1 cup bok choy
> 1 cup spinach
> ½ cup celery
> ½ cup carrots
> ½ cup fresh tomato
> ½ cup natural Parmesan cheese
> 2 ounces almonds, sliced

Dressing

> ½ cup plain yogurt
> 1 teaspoon rosemary
> 1 teaspoon honey
> 1 tablespoon lime juice
> Dash garlic powder

To make:

Rinse the salad greens, and pat dry. In a large bowl tear the greens into bite-size pieces, and toss. Thinly slice the carrots, then chop the celery, and tomatoes; put all on top of the greens. Add the cheese and almonds; lightly toss. Make the dressing by combining all the ingredients in a small bowl. Stir until blended, and pour over salad. Makes 4 servings.

Variations:

- Substitute napa cabbage for one of the greens.
- Substitute 1 cup fresh basil for one of the greens.
- Add 1 slice cucumber and ½ cup bean sprouts.
- Add 3 tablespoons chopped sun-dried tomatoes.
- Add one 11-ounce can of drained mandarin oranges.

31. Grilled Veggie Salad

You need:

>
> 1 red pepper
> 1 green pepper
> 1 yellow pepper
> 1 large onion
> 6 ounces mushrooms
> 1 cup Italian or balsamic vinegar
> dressing
> 1 teaspoon onion powder
> 1 teaspoon Salt Free Garlic and
> Herb Seasoning (McCormick)
> 4 cups romaine lettuce
> 2 ounces Gorgonzola cheese,
> crumbled

To make:

You need a vegetable tray for the grill, which can be purchased at most garden shops. Light the grill about 10 minutes before cooking. Cut peppers and onion into ⅜-inch strips. Purchase sliced mushrooms or slice ¼-inch thick. Place all veggies in a large zipper plastic bag with 1 cup of dressing. (You can also do this in a large covered bowl and marinate overnight in the refrigerator.) Drain liquid, and place vegetables on grilling tray. Grill veggies until brown on the edges or desired tenderness (about 20 to 30 minutes), checking and turning every 5 to 10 minutes. To grill in the oven, place vegetables on a baking sheet and broil on low about 5″ from heat for up to ½ hour; check and turn every 5 to 10 minutes until done. You can double the recipe and keep some for the next day as they marinate and are delicious. To serve, clean, and divide the romaine lettuce among four plates. Top with vegetables and Gorgonzola cheese. Makes 4 servings.

Variations:

- Add other favorite vegetables such as sliced yellow squash, zucchini, and eggplant. Modify amount of dressing with the additional vegetables.
- Substitute natural grated Parmesan cheese for Gorgonzola.

Doctor's ℞: Are you getting enough calcium to prevent bone loss? Check out the latest requirements:

Infants: 0 to 6 months, 210 milligrams; 6 to 12 months, 270 milligrams

Children: 1 to 3 years, 500 milligrams; 4 to 8 years, 800 milligrams; 9 to 18 years, 1,300 milligrams

Adults: 19 to 50 years, 1,000 milligrams; 51 and older, 1,500 milligrams

Pregnant and lactating women: 1,000 to 1,500 milligrams

32. Orange Fruit and Vanilla Cream

You need:

> 3 cups strawberries, stems
> removed
> 1 banana, sliced
> ½ cup apricots (fresh apricots—
> remove seeds, cut in half; canned
> apricots—drain, cut in half)
> 1 cup melon (use cantaloupe,
> honeydew, or watermelon, cut into
> bite-size pieces)
> 1 cup segments from 2 to 3 medium
> oranges
> 1 kiwi, peeled, sliced
> ¼ cup sweetened coconut
> ¼ cup orange juice

Dressing

> ½ cup fat-free or light sour cream
> 1½ cups fat-free or low-fat vanilla yogurt
> 3 tablespoons honey
> 1 vanilla bean (split open to expose seeds)

To make:

In a large clear glass compote (or in single-serving parfait glasses), layer the fruit in the order above, topping with kiwi and coconut. Pour orange juice over the fruit (or 1 tablespoon over each parfait). Cover, and marinate fruit for several hours. To make the dressing: In a small bowl combine sour cream, yogurt, honey, and vanilla bean. Cover, and marinate for several hours. Stir again, and remove the vanilla bean. The seeds from the bean will remain in the dressing and add a rich vanilla flavor. Top each parfait with the dressing. Makes 6 to 8 servings.

Variations:

- Substitute the following bone-boosting fruit according to what is in season: papaya (peeled, and cut into bite-size pieces); mango (peeled, and cut into bite-size pieces); tangerine segments; raspberries; blueberries; or blackberries.
- Top fruit with 2 tablespoons of chopped cashews, or divide among individual servings.
- Substitute 3 teaspoons vanilla flavoring for vanilla bean.

Chef's Comments: Consider egg substitutes over fresh eggs if you need a boost in vitamin A. Four ounces of egg substitutes have 1200 IUs of vitamin A while two eggs have 617 IUs.

33. Orange Jicama Salad

You need:

> 4 cups fresh spinach, cleaned,
>   patted dry
> 1 16-ounce jicama
> 2 large onions
> 2 tablespoons red onion, chopped
> ¼ cup sunflower seeds

Dressing

> ½ cup orange juice
> 1 tablespoon extra light olive oil

To make:

Arrange spinach on 4 individual plates. Peel the jicama, and cut into ¼-inch strips; divide equally among four plates. Peel and cut oranges into segments, then divide among the plates. Put some red onions and sunflower seeds on top of each salad. To make vinaigrette: In a small bowl combine orange juice and olive oil and whisk, pouring over each salad. Makes 4 servings.

34. Parmesan Sweet Basil and Bow Tie Salad

You need:

>   3 cups bow tie pasta, uncooked
>   1 red pepper, finely chopped
>   1 green pepper, finely chopped
>   ½ cup black olives
>   4 tablespoons green onions
>   2 tablespoons sweet basil (fresh)
>   Salt and pepper to taste

Dressing

>   3 tablespoons extra light olive oil
>   2 limes
>   1 tablespoon Parmesan cheese
>   Dash garlic powder
>   Extra Parmesan cheese for topping on salad
>   (optional)

To make:

Cook the pasta according to directions on package; cool under ice water, and drain. In a medium bowl, combine pasta, red pepper, green pepper, olives, onions, sweet basil, and salt and pepper. To make dressing: Combine olive oil, the juice of the limes, Parmesan cheese, and garlic powder. Pour over salad and serve. Top with additional Parmesan cheese to taste (optional). Makes 4 servings.

Variation:

-   Grate ½ teaspoon lime zest over salad before tossing with dressing.

35. Spinach Gorgonzola Salad

You need:

> 6 cups fresh spinach (clean, pat
> dry, and tear into bite-size
> pieces)
> 1 hard-boiled egg, chopped
> 2 ounces Gorgonzola cheese
> ½ green onion
> ¼ cup dry roasted cashews,
> chopped

Dressing

> 2 ounces Gorgonzola cheese
> ¼ cup fat-free or light sour cream
> 1 tablespoon white wine vinegar
> Dash Salt Free Garlic and Herb Seasoning
> (McCormick)
> ½ teaspoon curry powder

To make:

Put torn spinach in a large salad bowl, and top with the chopped boiled egg and chopped green onions. Cover with 2 ounces of Gorgonzola cheese. To make dressing: In a small microwave-proof bowl, put 2 ounces Gorgonzola cheese. Microwave for 30 seconds; stir in sour cream, and microwave for 30 more seconds. Add vinegar and stir. Pour over salad, then top with chopped cashews. Makes 6 servings.

Variations:

- Substitute grated Parmesan for Gorgonzola. Do not microwave until you mix this into the sour cream.

36. Tabouli Salad

You need:

> 1 cup bulgur wheat, fine
> 1 bunch green onions, with tops
> 1½ tablespoon finely chopped mint
>   leaves
> 2 large bunches parsley
> 4 medium tomatoes
> ⅓ cup lemon juice
> ½ cup extra light olive oil
> Salt and pepper to taste

To make:

Pour bulgur wheat into a large bowl, and cover with cold water 1 to 1½ hours or until softened. Drain in a colander that has cheesecloth or several paper towels layered on the bottom. Squeeze dry. Chop green onions, mint leaves, parsley without stems, and tomatoes very fine, or use a food processor (chopper blade), then put all ingredients in a large salad bowl. Add lemon juice, olive oil, and salt and pepper and mix well. Add more salt and pepper, if needed. Makes 6 to 8 servings.

Doctor's ℞: Giving your family high-calcium but low-fat foods such as skim milk, low-fat milk, low-fat cheeses, nonfat yogurt, and calcium-enriched juices and breads, along with calcium supplements, can make it easy for a weight-conscious teenager to get the necessary 1,300 mg of calcium each day.

———————

37. Waldorf Salad in Papaya Shell

You need:

- ½ cup fat-free or low-fat plain yogurt
- 1 tablespoon fat-free or low-fat mayonnaise
- 1 tablespoon orange juice
- 1 tablespoon honey
- Dash salt
- 3 papayas, 1 chopped for filling and 2 for shells (if out of season, use melons or oranges)
- ¾ cup celery, chopped
- 3 red apples, chopped with skin
- ¼ cup golden currants
- ½ cup cashews, chopped

To make:

To make dressing: In a small bowl, combine yogurt, mayonnaise, orange juice, honey, and salt. To make salad: Peel 1 papaya, and cut into bite-size pieces. In a large bowl, mix papaya, celery, apples, currants, and cashews. Add dressing to fruit, and stir well. Cut the remaining papayas in half, clean out seeds, and cut a thin slice off the bottom so the shell sits flat on the plate. If out of season, use melon or orange shells. Fill shells with salad. Makes 4 servings.

Chef's Comments: Spices can be bone-boosting, too! One tablespoon of oregano has 73 mg of calcium, and one teaspoon of paprika has 1273 IUs of vitamin A.

Sauces

38. Béchamel Sauce (thick white sauce)

You need:

> 3 tablespoons butter
> 4 tablespoons flour
> 2 cups fat-free or low-fat calcium-
> fortified milk
> ¼ teaspoon nutmeg
> Salt and white pepper to taste

To make:

In a heavy saucepan, melt butter on medium heat. Stir in flour, and cook for 1 minute, stirring constantly. Slowly add milk and continue to stir so that lumps do not form; add nutmeg, salt, and white pepper. Cook for 5 to 8 minutes, stirring constantly to keep the sauce from sticking. Use immediately over pasta or vegetables. Or cover, and use later. Makes 4 servings.

Variation:

- For a thinner sauce, add ¼ cup milk. To thicken, decrease milk by ⅛ to ¼ cup.
- Add ¼ cup nonfat dried milk to increase bone-boosting calcium.
- Add ¼ cup of your favorite cheese and ¼ cup fresh herbs, such as cilantro or basil.

39. Fresh Basil and Creamy Parmesan Sauce

You need:

> 2 cups béchamel sauce (see page 208)
> ½ cup fat-free or low-fat calcium-fortified milk
> ½ cup natural Parmesan cheese, grated
> Dash nutmeg
> 1 cup fresh sweet basil
> ¼ cup herbs of choice (try a combination of parsley, chives, cilantro, or oregano)
> Dash salt

To make:

In a heavy sauce pan, make béchamel sauce according to the directions, adding an additional ½ cup of milk. When sauce starts to thicken, add Parmesan cheese, nutmeg, basil, and herbs. Cook 5 to 10 minutes longer or until the sauce thickens. Adjust to taste with salt and pepper, and serve over your favorite pasta or vegetables. Makes 4 to 6 servings.

40. Tomato and Fresh Basil Sauce

You need:

>3 cloves garlic, chopped
>1 white onion, finely chopped
>⅓ extra light olive oil
>5 large tomatoes, chopped into
>   bite-size pieces
>2 teaspoons sugar
>1 tablespoon fresh sweet basil
>Salt and pepper to taste
>½ cup Parmesan cheese, fresh,
>   grated

To make:

In a large saucepan, cook garlic and onion over medium-high heat in olive oil until onion pieces are clear and soft. Reduce heat to medium, and add tomatoes, sugar, and basil; salt and pepper to taste. Cook an additional 15 minutes, and stir occasionally. Serve over your favorite pasta, and top with Parmesan. For an elegant presentation, add more basil over dish before serving. Makes 4 servings.

Variations:

- Grate a teaspoon of lime, lemon, or orange into pasta sauce when you add tomatoes for a crisp clean taste.

Main Dishes

BEEF

41. Beef and Chicken Medley

You need:

> 2 chicken breasts, skinned,
> debound
> 2 pounds sirloin tips
> 1 cup sherry
> ¼ cup extra light olive oil
> 1 onion, finely chopped
> ½ teaspoon salt
> ½ teaspoon pepper
> ½ teaspoon Salt Free Garlic and
> Herb Seasoning (McCormick)
> 2 bay leaves
> ½ cup tomato paste
> 2 cups low-sodium beef bouillon or
> broth
> 2 carrots, finely chopped
> 10 ounces frozen spinach
> 2 cups brown basmati rice
> (prepared according to
> directions)

To make:

Cut chicken into ½ inch strips and beef into 1-inch cubes. Marinate chicken and beef in sherry, olive oil, onion, and spices (salt, pepper, Garlic and Herb, and bay leaves). You can prepare this the night before, and let marinate in the refrigerator overnight. Or marinate at least several hours for fuller flavor if you plan to use it the same day. Put meat, marinade, tomato paste, and bouillon in a large heavy pot, and cook over medium heat for 2 hours. Add carrots, celery, and spinach, and continue to cook for another 45 minutes, checking beef for tenderness every 15 minutes. Slowly increase heat for 10 to 15 minutes to thicken the sauce, stirring frequently. Adjust seasoning with salt and pepper. Serve over brown basmati rice which has been prepared according to directions. (Basmati rice is a long-grained rice with a nutlike flavor and aroma and is found in Indian and Middle Eastern markets and most supermarkets.) Makes 6 servings.

Doctor's ℞: It is not too late to keep bones strong in later adult years, though many women begin to experience fractures shortly after menopause due to the drastic decline of estrogen and this injurious result on bone mass. After this life change, women should increase their calcium intake to 1,500 mg each day between diet and supplements. The average diet after menopause contains 800 mg of calcium. In fact, studies have shown that 80 percent of all postmenopausal women do not get adequate calcium to stop bone loss.

———————

42. Beef Stroganoff

You need:

> 3 pounds beef filet, defatted, cut
>   into 1″ cubes
> ½ teaspoon salt (or salt substitute)
> 1 teaspoon pepper
> 1 teaspoon Salt Free Garlic and
>   Herb Seasoning (McCormick)
> 1 teaspoon nutmeg
> 3 tablespoons flour
> 1 stick of reduced-calorie
>   margarine (or regular)
> 2 tablespoons extra light olive oil
> 3 cups low-sodium beef bouillon or
>   broth
> 2 cups béchamel sauce (page 208)
> 8 ounces fat-free or light sour
>   cream
> 2 tablespoons Dijon mustard
> 3 tablespoons Worcestershire
>   sauce
> 1 teaspoon paprika
> 1 white onion, finely chopped
> 8 ounces white mushrooms, sliced
> 2 tablespoons fresh parsley

To make:

To prepare meat, cut all visible fat off of beef, then slice into 1-inch cubes. Put ½ teaspoon each of salt, pepper, Salt Free Garlic and Herb Seasoning, nutmeg, and flour over the meat. Using a large heavy pot, sauté half of the beef in 2 tablespoons margarine and 1 tablespoon olive oil. When this is lightly browned, sauté the other half of the beef cubes in 2 tablespoons margarine and 1 tablespoon olive oil. Add bouillon and cook for 1½ hours over medium heat, or until beef is tender to cut. (This time may vary according to the quality of the beef you are using.) Prepare béchamel sauce (white sauce) according to the directions given on page 208.

In a medium sauce pan, add béchamel sauce, sour cream, Dijon mustard, Worcestershire sauce, paprika, and ½ teaspoon each of the Garlic and Herb, pepper, and nutmeg. Simmer this for 10 minutes on low heat, then remove pan from heat while meat continues to cook. Chop the onion in fine pieces, then sauté onion in 2 tablespoons margarine until clear; add to white sauce mixture. Wash and dry mushrooms, cutting the end of the stems off. Cut the mushrooms into thin slices. Sauté the mushrooms until golden in 2 tablespoons margarine, and add to white sauce mixture. Just before serving this dish, prepare your favorite noodles. Have a large pasta plate or casserole dish available. Drain pasta, then using a slotted spoon, put meat without bouillon over pasta, reserving 1 cup bouillon or beef sauce. Pour 1 cup bouillon or beef sauce into the white sauce, stir well, then pour this over beef and pasta. Sprinkle parsley generously over the entire stroganoff and plate to decorate. Serve immediately. Makes 6 servings.

Chef's Comments: A bone-boosting dessert can be made out of leftover sweet potatoes (peeled and sliced), sliced apples and bananas, chopped dates, and chopped dried apricots. Add such favorite nuts as almonds, walnuts, cashews, peanuts, Brazil nuts, pumpkin seeds, grated toasted coconut, honey, and citrus juices (lime, lemon, or orange). Mix and match your favorites, adding honey and citrus to suit your taste.

———————————

43. Southern Italian Meatballs

You need:

>   3 slices bread (calcium-fortified)
>   2 pounds ground sirloin
>   1 onion, finely chopped
>   ¼ cup Parmesan cheese, grated
>   ¼ cup silken tofu
>   2 tablespoons catsup
>   ½ teaspoon Salt Free Garlic and
>   Herb Seasoning (McCormick)
>   1 tablespoon oregano
>   ½ teaspoon salt
>   ½ teaspoon pepper
>   Cooking spray

To make:

Preheat oven to 400 degrees. Place bread in the blender, and blend to make crumbs. In a large bowl, mix ground sirloin, onion, Parmesan cheese, tofu, catsup, bread crumbs, Salt Free Garlic and Herb Seasoning, oregano, salt, and pepper. When mixture is combined, form into 1-inch balls, and place on a baking sheet coated with cooking spray. Bake about 20 minutes, or until brown and crispy. Drain excess oil, and serve over favorite pasta topped with Sweet Tomato Cream sauce (page 264). Makes about 3 dozen small meatballs.

POULTRY

44. Chicken Cacciatore

You need:

- 4 boneless, skinless chicken breasts
- ½ teaspoon salt
- 1 teaspoon white pepper
- 4 tablespoons extra light olive oil
- 2 onions, finely chopped
- 3 cloves garlic
- 2 red peppers
- ½ cup white wine
- 1 tablespoon fresh basil
- 1 16-ounce can Italian plum tomatoes
- ½ teaspoon sugar
- 2 tablespoons fresh parsley

To make:

Sprinkle chicken with ½ teaspoon salt and ½ teaspoon pepper, then in a large sauce pan on medium-high heat, sauté chicken in olive oil until golden brown. Move chicken to one side of the pan, and add onions, garlic, and red peppers. Sauté for 3 to 4 minutes until light brown. Add wine, ½ teaspoon pepper, basil, and tomatoes to the chicken-onion mixture. Simmer on medium heat for 20 minutes, breaking apart the tomatoes. Add sugar. Serve with pasta or rice; sprinkle fresh parsley over the entire plate. Makes 4 servings.

45. Chicken and Broccoli with Creamy Sun-Dried Tomato Sauce

You need:

> 1 14-ounce bag frozen broccoli
> florets
> 4 boneless, skinless chicken breasts
> 1 garlic clove
> 2 tablespoons extra light olive oil
> Salt and pepper
> 15 to 20 sun-dried tomatoes,
> chopped
> ¾ cup fresh basil, chopped
> ¾ cup fat-free or low-fat calcium-
> fortified milk
> ½ fat-free or low-fat sour cream
> ½ cup Romano or Parmesan cheese

To make:

Cook broccoli according to directions; drain and set aside. In a large sauce pan, sauté chicken and garlic in olive oil on medium-high until golden on both sides and cooked through. Add sun-dried tomatoes, and continue cooking for another minute. Add ½ cup basil, milk, sour cream, and ½ teaspoon salt and ½ teaspoon pepper. Continue to cook sauce until it starts to thicken; add broccoli. Pour into a serving dish. Sprinkle cheese and ¼ cup basil over entire dish for a beautiful presentation. Serve over your favorite rice or pasta. Makes 4 to 6 servings.

Variation:

- Grate ½ teaspoon of citrus zest into sauce while thickening.

46. Chicken and Yellow Rice

You need:

>4 boneless, skinless chicken
>   breasts, cut in half lengthwise
>3 tablespoons extra light olive oil
>Salt and pepper
>1 large onion, chopped
>1 red pepper, chopped
>1 green bell pepper, chopped
>2 garlic cloves
>1 teaspoon onion powder
>2 bay leaves
>4 cups water
>1 16-ounce can diced tomatoes with
>   liquid
>1 10-ounce package Vigo Yellow
>   Rice with spices
>1 can tiny green peas, drained

To make:

Preheat oven to 350 degrees. Using a frying pan, sauté chicken in olive oil on medium-high heat for several minutes on each side. Add onion, then peppers and garlic. Continue to sauté the chicken until the onions and peppers are soft. Add spices, ½ teaspoon salt, ½ teaspoon pepper, water, and tomatoes including juice. Bring to a boil, then add rice and spices included in package. Boil for one minute, stir, then pour into a 4-quart baking dish. Top with drained peas, and cover with foil. Bake for 45 minutes in the center of the oven. After 30 minutes, check the edges and make sure the rice is moist but not wet. If you overcook and rice is dry along the edges, add ½ cup water and bake 10 more minutes. If the sides of the rice are showing liquid, cook another 5 minutes, and test again. Serve with crispy bread and Feta Cabbage Salad (page 197). Makes 6 to 8 servings.

Doctor's ℞: Stopping cigarette smoking and cutting back on alcohol are prevention measures you hold in your own hands—literally! In fact, the risk of osteoporosis drops in half when you stop smoking. The chances of having heart disease, cancer, stroke, or emphysema also decrease upon quitting.

———————

47. Curried Chicken and Fruit Salad

You need:

>   ½ teaspoon onion powder
>   ½ teaspoon garlic powder
>   ½ teaspoon curry
>   1 bay leaf
>   1 whole chicken
>   ½ cup dates, chopped
>   ⅓ cup yellow currants
>   1 golden delicious apple, sliced with
>   peel
>   ¼ cup slivered almonds
>   Dash salt and pepper
>   ⅓ cup toasted coconut
>   3 cups romaine lettuce, shredded
>   Paprika

Dressing:

>   ¾ cup fat-free or light sour cream
>   ¼ cup fat-free or low-fat mayonnaise
>   ¼ teaspoon salt and white pepper
>   ½ teaspoon curry powder (can use up to 1
>   teaspoon for a more flavorful dish)
>   ¼ cup crushed pineapple in its own juices

To make:

In a large pot, add 2 cups of water, onion powder, garlic powder, curry, and the bay leaf. Poach the chicken in this for 30 minutes or until done. Cool the chicken, and pull off the meat, putting this into a large bowl. (You can freeze the chicken broth for other recipes that need low-sodium bouillon.) Add the dates, currants, sliced apple, almond slivers, and dash of salt and pepper. Broil the coconut for 1 minute, or until it starts to turn light brown. In a small bowl, combine sour cream, mayonnaise, salt and pepper, curry powder, and crushed pineapple. Spoon chicken mixture onto shredded romaine, and top with dressing. Sprinkle toasted coconut over the sauce, then sprinkle with paprika. Makes 4 to 6 servings.

Chef's Comments: Sesame seeds are easy to add to salads, breads, dips, and vegetables. One ounce of sesame seeds has 160 calories, 281 mg of calcium, and 101 mg of magnesium.

—————————

48. Mandarin Chicken

You need:

> Salt and pepper
> 4 chicken breasts
> 2 tablespoons olive oil (optional, if sautéing)
> 1 8-ounce can diced water chestnuts
> ¾ cup celery, sliced
> ⅓ slivered almonds (reserve 1 tablespoon for garnish)
> ¾ cup chunk pineapple in own juices, drained
> ¾ cup green grapes (reserve several grapes per serving for garnish)
> 2 8-ounce cans mandarin oranges, drained (reserve ¼ cup orange segments for garnish)
> ¼ cup golden raisins
> ¼ cups romaine lettuce, shredded

Dressing:

> 1 cup fat-free or light sour cream
> ½ cup fat-free or low-fat mayonnaise
> 1 tablespoon extra light olive oil
> ½ teaspoon citrus zest (grate orange, lemon or lime zest over dressing)
> ½ teaspoon grated ginger
> Salt and white pepper to taste

To make:

Salt and pepper chicken breasts, then boil or sauté in olive oil until thoroughly cooked. Cool, then dice into bite-size pieces. In a large bowl, combine chicken, water chestnuts, celery, almonds, pineapples, grapes, oranges, and raisins. Prepare dressing in a small bowl by mixing sour cream, mayonnaise, olive oil, citrus zest, and ginger. Adjust dressing with salt and white pepper to taste. Serve over a bed of romaine lettuce. Top with the dressing, and garnish with several grapes or oranges and a few almonds. Makes 6 servings.

Variations:

- Substitute ½ cup softened tofu for ½ cup light sour cream.

49. White Wine Chicken and Shrimp Newberg

You need:

> 4 boneless, skinless chicken breasts
> 3 tablespoons olive oil
> ½ teaspoon salt and pepper
> 2 cups of assorted fresh seasonal
>   vegetables, such as:
>   peas, shelled
>   broccoli florets
>   cauliflower florets
>   cabbage, chopped
>   carrots, thinly sliced
>   potatoes, thinly sliced
>   green beans
>   spinach
>   leeks, chopped
> ½ cup mushrooms, sliced
> 2 tablespoons flour
> 8 ounces white wine
> 8 ounces low-sodium vegetable or
>   chicken broth
> ¼ teaspoon thyme
> ½ teaspoon garlic
> ¼ teaspoon nutmeg
> 1 pound large shrimp, peeled,
>   deveined, no tails
> 1 cup asparagus
> 1 15-ounce can plum tomatoes, cut
>   into quarters
> 1 tablespoon fresh basil
> 1 tablespoon fresh parsley

To make:

In a medium-size saucepan, sauté chicken in olive oil until brown on both sides. Put the chicken in a heavy 3-quart pot, and add assorted vegetables to the chicken; salt and pepper. Using the pan you cooked the chicken in, sauté mushrooms in the olive oil, cooking until brown. Add flour to the mushrooms, and cook for a minute. Slowly add wine and broth while stirring. Continue to cook until sauce begins to thicken, or about 5 to 6 minutes. Transfer the mushrooms and sauce to the pot with the chicken and vegetables. Add thyme, garlic, and nutmeg. Cook for 20 minutes on medium-low heat. Add shrimp, asparagus, tomato, basil, and parsley. Cook another 15 minutes. Serve with baked potato. Makes 6 servings.

SEAFOOD
50. Ginger Salmon Florentine

You need:

    4 salmon steaks (about 8 ounces each, cut
        ¾" thick)
    1 tablespoon low-sodium soy sauce
    1 tablespoon Worcestershire sauce
    Dash garlic powder
    1 teaspoon fresh ginger, peeled, grated
    1 cup béchamel sauce (page 208)
    2 10-ounce packages frozen spinach
    ½ teaspoon dry mustard
    1½ cup Gruyère cheese (reserve ½ cup for
        topping)
    1 lime (cut into quarters)
    2 cups favorite pasta, prepared

To make:

Put salmon steaks in a large plastic bag, and set aside. In a small bowl, mix soy sauce, Worcestershire sauce, garlic, and ginger. Pour liquid over steaks, and marinate in the refrigerator for 1 hour. Turn several times. Cook spinach according to directions, drain, and pat dry. In a medium saucepan, cook ½ recipe of béchamel sauce on page 208. Add spinach, dry mustard, and 1 cup Gruyère cheese. Cook for several minutes, melting cheese. Take the pan off the heat, and set aside. Preheat the broiler, and set the rack on the top shelf or about 4 to 5 inches from the broiler. On a large baking sheet, broil the steaks for about 8 minutes on each side, basting as you turn the steaks. The steaks should appear opaque when tested with the tip of a knife. The cooking time will depend on the temperature of your oven and the distance from the broiler. Meanwhile, spoon the creamy spinach into a 2-quart greased casserole dish. Top this with the salmon steaks and ½ cup Gruyère cheese. Broil for one minute to melt cheese and serve. Place a lime wedge on each plate, and serve with favorite pasta. Makes 4 servings.

51. Linguine and Salmon Italian

You need:

> 1 onion, chopped
> 2 tablespoons extra light olive oil
> 2 7.5-ounce cans of salmon,
>   drained
> ½ teaspoon Salt Free Garlic and
>   Herb Seasoning (McCormick)
> 1 14.5-ounce can chunky tomatoes
> ¼ teaspoon salt
> ¼ teaspoon pepper
> 3 tablespoons fresh basil (or 1
>   tablespoon dried basil)
> 1 tablespoon lime juice
> 1 16-ounce package of linguine
> ½ cup natural Parmesan cheese,
>   grated
> 1 tablespoon parsley

To make:

In a medium sauce pan, sauté chopped onion in olive oil on medium-high heat until clear. Add drained salmon, and continue to cook for several minutes longer. To the onion-salmon mixture, add Salt Free Garlic and Herb Seasoning, tomatoes, salt, pepper, basil, and lime juice. Cook for 10 more minutes. Cover, then remove from heat while you prepare the linguine according to package instructions. Drain linguine and place on a serving platter, topping with sauce. Sprinkle Parmesan cheese over the top, then sprinkle parsley over the entire platter. Makes 4 to 6 servings.

Doctor's ℞: While the calcium needs of vegans are not fully understood, studies have found that vegans may actually need less calcium than their meat-eating contemporaries. This could be because of the negative affect animal protein has on calcium absorption in the body. If you are a vegetarian, choose such calcium-rich foods as legumes, calcium-fortified juices, soy nuts, calcium-fortified soy milk, and molasses. Also make sure to eat such vegetables as artichokes, broccoli, brussels sprouts, cabbage, carrots, celery, lima beans, snap beans, spinach, and Swiss chard.

———————————

52. Mandarin Orange Shrimp in a Papaya

You need:

- ½ cup orange juice
- ½ cup water
- 2 pounds of shrimp, shelled, deveined
- ½ cup fat-free or light sour cream
- ¼ cup fat-free or light mayonnaise
- 1 teaspoon orange zest (page 278)
- 1 5-ounce can diced water chestnuts
- ½ cup celery, chopped
- ½ cup green onions, chopped
- 1 11-ounce can mandarin oranges, drained
- 2 papaya, cut in half, seeds removed (use orange or melon shell, depending on season)
- 1 tablespoon fresh chives (or parsley)

To make:

In a medium sauce pan, heat orange juice and water on medium high, then add shrimp. Boil for about 10 minutes or until shrimp is pink. In a colander, drain shrimp and cool with ice water. Put drained shrimp in a medium-sized bowl. In a small bowl combine sour cream, mayonnaise, orange zest, water chestnuts, celery, and green onions. Pour over shrimp, stir well, and add oranges. Cut the two papayas into halves, removing seeds, then cut a thin slice off the bottom of each papaya half, so fruit will sit flat on plate. Put one-fourth of shrimp mixture in each papaya, and top with fresh chives. Makes 4 servings.

Chef's Comments: Textured vegetable protein (TVP) has a similar isoflavone profile as the soybean. TVP is a common filler for casseroles and burgers with 138.2 isoflavones per cup.

53. Shrimp and Vegetables in Sherry Cream

You need:

> ½ cup margarine (or reduced-
> calorie margarine)
> 1 onion, chopped
> 1 celery stalk, chopped
> 1 carrot, chopped
> 8 ounces mushrooms, sliced
> 2 pounds large shrimp, cleaned,
> deveined, without tails
> 1 tablespoon lemon juice
> ⅓ cup sherry
> 2 cups béchamel sauce (page 208)
> Salt and pepper to taste
> 3 cups rice (prepared according to
> directions)

To make:

In a large saucepan, melt ¼ cup margarine (reserve the remaining margarine for later) on medium high, then sauté onion, celery, and carrot until onion pieces are clear and carrot pieces are almost cooked through (about 5 minutes). Add mushrooms, and continue cooking for 3 to 4 minutes. Add shrimp and lemon juice, and cook 10 minutes. Turn heat down to medium before vegetables turn brown. Stir in sherry, and cook several minutes longer. Add béchamel sauce, and stir in remaining margarine; add salt and pepper to taste. Prepare rice of your choice, and serve shrimp and vegetables over the rice. Makes 6 servings.

54. Smoked Salmon with Ginger Vinaigrette

You need:

> 4 cups fresh spinach, rinsed, patted dry
> 1 5-ounce can sliced water chestnuts, drained
> ⅓ cup walnuts, chopped
> 1 tablespoon parsley
> ⅓ pound smoked salmon, sliced into 8 strips
> 1 orange, cut into four segments, about ¼-inch thick, including rind to use for decoration (save the rest of the orange for vinaigrette and orange zest)

Vinaigrette

> 4 tablespoons orange juice
> ½ teaspoon orange zest (page 278)
> ½ teaspoon sugar
> 3 tablespoons light olive oil
> 2-inch piece ginger, grated

To make:

In a large bowl, combine spinach, water chestnuts, walnuts, and parsley. Put on four individual plates, and top with 2 slices of salmon on each plate. To make the vinaigrette: In a medium bowl, combine freshly squeezed orange juice, zest, sugar, and olive oil. Grate ginger to make 2 teaspoons, add to dressing, and whisk the dressing well. Pour vinaigrette over the salmon and spinach, and top with a slice of orange for decoration. Makes 4 servings.

Soups
55. Chilled Pineapple Gazpacho

You need:

> 1 large pineapple, peeled, cut into
>   chunks (or 2 cans pineapple
>   chunks in juice)
> ¼ cup fresh mint, chopped
> 1 large red onion, finely chopped
> 1 large green pepper, finely
>   chopped
> 1 large red pepper, finely chopped
> 1 cup fat-free or low-fat calcium-
>   fortified plain yogurt

To make:

In a food processor, puree pineapple chunks until smooth. Add fresh mint and blend. Stir in red onion and green and red peppers. Chill for four hours; serve with a dollop of plain yogurt and mint leaf on top. Makes 6 servings.

56. Creamy Butternut Squash Soup

You need:

> 4 tablespoons extra light olive oil
> 3 onions, chopped (or 12 ounces frozen chopped onions)
> 8 large potatoes, peeled, chopped
> 1 tablespoon onion powder
> 1 tablespoon Salt Free Garlic and Herb Seasoning (McCormick)
> Salt and pepper, to taste
> 8 cups water
> 1 package dehydrated onion soup mix
> 3 packages frozen butternut squash
> 3 cans chickpeas, drained, rinsed
> 2 cups evaporated skim milk
> 1 cup dehydrated potatoes (for thickening soup)

To make:

Pour olive oil in a large skillet, and sauté onions until soft. Add potatoes, stirring continually while adding onion powder, Salt Free Garlic and Herb Seasoning, and salt and pepper to taste. Add 8 cups water and dehydrated onion soup mix, continue to cook for about 20 minutes to soften potatoes. Drop butternut squash into soup, and stir until it is thawed. Add drained chickpeas, evaporated skim milk, dehydrated potatoes. Cook 20 minutes longer, and adjust spices to taste. Serves 10 to 12.

Variations:

- If time allows, cook dried chickpeas to cut down on the sodium.
- Make a large batch of soup, then divide into three or four containers. Freeze for an instant bone-boosting addition to a quick sandwich or salad.

- Put a dollop of reduced-calorie or nonfat sour cream on top with a sprig of cilantro.

Doctor's ℞: Watch your daughter's diet! An article published in the January 1997 issue of the Journal of Adolescent Health reported that only 2 percent of girls ages 15 to 18 in the United States get enough calcium to keep bones strong. Encourage all children to grab a milkshake at fast-food restaurants and order "extra cheese" on hamburgers. Keep string cheese on hand for quick after school snacks, and whip up a fruit and yogurt smoothie as a bedtime treat.

———————

57. Healthy Vegetable Broth

You need:

> 4 stalks celery, chopped
> 4 carrots, chopped
> 1 onion, chopped
> 1 garlic clove
> ½ cup parsley
> ½ cup fresh herbs of choice (basil, oregano, or chives)
> ½ teaspoon Salt Free Garlic and Herb Seasoning (McCormick)
> ½ teaspoon onion powder
> ¼ teaspoon salt (optional)
> ½ teaspoon pepper
> ½ cup greens of choice (spinach, turnips, or collards)
> 6 cups water

To make:

In a large soup pot combine all ingredients, and simmer for 20 minutes. Cool and refrigerate, or freeze for a low-sodium bone-boosting broth. Can be substituted in any recipe for bouillon or broth. Strain vegetables out if you need a clear broth.

Chef's Comments: Substitute natural Parmesan cheese for Gorgonzola and reduce fat by 5 grams and calories by 60. Go one step further and use fat-free Parmesan or mozzarella cheese in recipes that call for cheese.

———————

58. Red, White, and Green Soup

You need:

>   1 large onion, chopped
>   2 tablespoons extra light olive oil
>   ½ cup leeks, chopped
>   1 green bell pepper, cut into ¼-inch
>   strips
>   2 pounds of red potatoes, chopped
>   with peel
>   4 cups vegetarian low-sodium
>   broth (low-sodium bouillon or
>   broth may be substituted)
>   1 teaspoon Mrs. Dash
>   ½ teaspoon Salt Free Garlic and
>   Herb Seasoning (McCormick)
>   1 teaspoon onion powder
>   ½ teaspoon pepper
>   4 cups mustard greens (spinach or
>   collards may be substituted),
>   washed, shredded
>   ½ cup fat-free or light sour cream
>   ¼ cup fresh cilantro or parsley for
>   decoration (optional)

To make:

In a large soup pot, sauté chopped onion and leeks for 2 to 3 minutes on medium-high heat in olive oil. When onion is clear and soft, add pepper strips. Cook for several minutes longer. Add red potatoes to vegetables. Add broth and spices, turn temperature down to medium-low, and simmer. Cook for 20 minutes, then add favorite seasonal greens. Steam for another 10 minutes. Let soup cool slightly. Serve with a dollop of light sour cream in the center of each bowl and a sprig of cilantro or parsley. Makes 6 to 8 servings.

Variations:

- Use a dash of paprika on the sour cream instead of the herbs.
- Sprinkle grated natural Parmesan over the sour cream.

Pasta and Rice Dishes
59. Cheesy Chicken Manicotti

You need:

> 12 manicotti shells, uncooked
> 1½ cups chicken breast, cooked,
>   cut in 1-inch chunks
> 1 cup wilted spinach, drained
> 1 cup fat-free or low-fat ricotta
>   cheese
> 2 tablespoons cilantro, fresh
> ¼ cup onion, chopped
> 2 cloves garlic, minced
> 1 cup fat-free spaghetti sauce or
>   marinara sauce
> ⅓ cup natural Parmesan cheese,
>   grated

To make:

Preheat oven to 325 degrees. Cook manicotti shells according to package directions. While shells are boiling, mix chicken breast, spinach, ricotta cheese, cilantro, onion, and garlic in a large bowl. Drain shells, then fill with chicken mixture. Place each shell in a 13×8-inch ungreased glass dish; pour spaghetti sauce over shells, then sprinkle with Parmesan cheese. Cover with lid or foil, and bake for 40 minutes. Makes 4 to 6 servings.

Variations:

- Substitute white meat turkey or lean beef for chicken breast.
- Substitute 1 cup grated zucchini or carrots for spinach.
- Use favorite cheese (Jack, feta, or Romano) instead of Parmesan.

60. Confetti Brown Rice

You need:

    2 tablespoons extra light olive oil
    1 cup calcium-fortified orange juice
    1½ cups water
    1 cup brown rice, uncooked
    1 pound medium shrimp, deveined, cut in half
    1 teaspoon fresh ginger, minced
    1 medium red onion, finely chopped
    2 cups fresh spinach, chopped, without stems
    ½ cup julienne carrots
    ½ cup green peas, frozen
    1 tablespoon low-sodium soy sauce
    ¼ teaspoon crushed red pepper flakes
    Salt to taste

To make:

In a 4-quart saucepan, heat 1 tablespoon olive oil, orange juice, and water, bringing this to a boil. Add the rice and stir. Reduce heat, cover the pan, and cook on medium low for 35 to 40 minutes. Fluff with a fork to separate; set aside. In a heavy skillet, heat 1 tablespoon oil over medium heat. Add ginger and onions. Using higher heat, add shrimp, and stir-fry for 4 minutes or until almost done. Add spinach, carrots, peas, soy sauce, and red pepper flakes to this; stir-fry for 4 more minutes. Salt to taste, remove from heat, and fold in rice. Makes 4 to 6 servings.

Variations:

- Substitute your favorite greens, such as kale, mustard, or collards.
- Add 10 chopped sun-dried tomatoes.
- Use boneless chicken or turkey breast strips instead of shrimp. Cook until done.

61. Creamy Broccoli and Sun-Dried Tomatoes on Bow Ties

You need:

> 2 cups béchamel sauce (page 208)
> 1 onion, finely chopped
> 2 tablespoons extra light olive oil
> 2 tablespoons sun-dried tomatoes, chopped
> 1 teaspoon fresh basil
> ½ cup almonds, sliced
> ½ teaspoon salt and pepper
> 1 16-ounce box bow tie pasta
> 1 pound frozen broccoli, chopped
> ½ cup fresh Romano cheese, grated

To make:

Prepare béchamel sauce (page 208); set aside. In a saucepan on medium-high heat, sauté onion in olive oil for 2 minutes, then add sun-dried tomatoes. Add béchamel sauce, basil, almonds, salt and pepper to saucepan. Cover saucepan and turn off heat. Cook pasta and broccoli separately, according to package directions. Drain pasta and broccoli in same colander, then spoon into a large pasta dish. Pour béchamel sauce and vegetables over pasta. Serve and top with fresh grated Romano cheese. Makes 6 to 8 servings.

Variations:

- Red peppers can be added or used instead of sun-dried tomatoes.
- Almonds can be replaced with chopped walnuts, water chestnuts, or jicama.
- 1 teaspoon of lime zest can be added to onion and sun-dried tomatoes when you are sautéing.
- Substitute frozen peas for broccoli.
- Sauté yellow squash and zucchini with onion and sun-dried tomatoes.

- Squeeze one lemon over broccoli and pasta before adding sauce.

Doctor's ℞: Serve a tall glass of calcium-fortified orange juice with your family's breakfast each morning. Not only will they get nearly one-third of their daily calcium requirement, but orange juice provides vitamin C and as much potassium as a banana.

---

62. Four Vegetables and Cheese Risotto

You need:

                1 large onion, finely chopped
                1 green bell pepper, chopped
                ½ teaspoon garlic powder
                2 tablespoons extra light olive oil
                6 cups water
                1 teaspoon rosemary
                1 bay leaf
                ½ teaspoon sage
                ½ teaspoon salt
                ½ teaspoon white pepper
                2 carrots, finely chopped
                2 cups white corn
                1 15-ounce can cut tomatoes,
                  undrained
                2 cups arborio (short-grain) rice,
                  cooked
                6 ounces goat cheese

To make:

In a large heavy pot, sauté onion, green bell pepper, and garlic powder in olive oil for 3 to 4 minutes. Add water, spices, salt, pepper, carrots, corn, and tomatoes, and cook for 8 to 10 minutes or until carrots are tender. Pour into a colander and catch vegetable broth to use in making rice or risotto. Risotto is an affectionate term for "rice" and means "little rice." Make risotto according to package instructions using the vegetable broth for the liquid. It should take about 30 minutes. When the risotto is done, stir in goat cheese and vegetables, then serve. Makes 8 servings.

Variations:

- Use instant white or brown rice to decrease cooking time.
- Substitute vegetables of choice.
- Cut a brick of tofu into 1-inch squares, and sauté with the onions and peppers.

Chef's Comments: Keep flavored chutneys and salsas on hand to add zest to bone-boosting salmon steaks. You can purchase these at specialty stores or check the gourmet section of your local supermarket for such interesting flavors as mango salsa.

———————

63. Fresh Basil al Pomodoro Bow Ties

You need:

>   2 tablespoons extra light olive oil
>   1 14-ounce can fresh cut tomatoes
>   1 teaspoon sugar
>   Salt and pepper to taste
>   2 tablespoons fresh basil
>   1 16-ounce box of bow tie pasta
>   ¾ cup natural Parmesan cheese,
>   grated

To make:

In a large sauce pan on medium-high heat, combine oil and tomatoes, mashing tomatoes while stirring. Cook for 8 to 10 minutes. Add sugar and salt and pepper to taste, then add whole basil leaves. (Fresh basil will give this dish a delicate flavor.) Continue to stir, reducing heat to low. Cook the pasta according to directions. Drain pasta, and put in a pasta serving bowl. Add sauce, and top with fresh grated Parmesan cheese. Makes 6 servings.

Variations:

• Add the juice of one orange, and stir in with tomatoes and oil.

64. Gorgonzola Spinach with Couscous

You need:

> 1 lemon (use 1 teaspoon lemon zest,
>   then save lemon juice)
> ¼ cup walnuts, chopped
> 2 cups fresh spinach, packed
> 1 tablespoon sun-dried tomatoes
> ½ teaspoon Salt Free Garlic and
>   Herb Seasoning (McCormick)
> 2 tablespoons extra light olive oil
> 1¼ cup low-sodium vegetable or
>   chicken broth
> 1 16-ounce can chickpeas, rinsed
>   and drained
> ½ teaspoon salt
> ½ teaspoon pepper
> ½ teaspoon onion powder
> 1 6-ounce package couscous
> ½ cup Gorgonzola, crumbled

To make:

Grate the lemon for 1 teaspoon of lemon zest; set aside. Toast walnuts in the microwave for 1 minute; set aside. In a medium saucepan, sauté the spinach and tomatoes with the Salt Free Garlic and Herb Seasoning and lemon zest in olive oil for several minutes or until spinach is wilted. Add broth and steam covered on low heat for 10 minutes. Add the chickpeas, salt, pepper, and onion powder. Bring mixture to a boil, and stir in couscous. Remove from heat, cover, and let stand for 5 minutes. Stir in 1 tablespoon reserved fresh lemon juice, Gorgonzola cheese, and walnuts. Makes 4 to 6 servings.

65. Penne Pasta and Roasted Vegetables

You need:

>   6 tomatoes (remove stem and cut into
>   4 to 6 pieces depending on the size
>   of the tomato)
>   3 cups broccoli florets
>   4 green onions, chopped
>   ½ cup vegetable broth
>   Dash Salt Free Garlic and Herb
>   Seasoning (McCormick)
>   8 ounces penne pasta
>   ½ teaspoon salt
>   ½ teaspoon pepper
>   2 tablespoons fresh basil, chopped
>   1 tablespoon white balsamic vinegar
>   2 tablespoons olive oil
>   ½ cup Romano cheese

To make:

Preheat oven to 425 degrees. Put tomatoes and broccoli florets in a 3-quart greased baking dish. Combine onions, vegetable broth, and Salt Free Garlic and Herb Seasoning, and pour over vegetables. Roast for 35 minutes, coating with broth several times. During the last 10 minutes of roasting the vegetables, cook the pasta according to directions, drain and pour into a pasta bowl or a serving platter. Check the roasted vegetables, making sure the broccoli is tender. Remove vegetables from the oven; add salt, pepper, and 1 tablespoon fresh basil (reserve the other tablespoon of basil for topping). Mix the balsamic vinegar and olive oil; pour over vegetables. Pour vegetables over pasta, and top with more fresh basil and Romano cheese. Makes 4 to 6 servings.

Vegetables

66. Carrots and Sweet Potatoes

You need:

> 1 16-ounce bag frozen carrots, sliced or
>   baby carrots
> 3 medium sweet potatoes
> 1 onion
> 1 tablespoon extra light olive oil
> 1 teaspoon sugar
> 2 cups fat-free or light sour cream
> ½ cup grated cheddar cheese (or reduced-
>   fat cheddar cheese)
> ½ cup sliced almonds (optional)

To make:

Preheat oven to 350 degrees. Place frozen carrots in a micro-wave-proof bowl. Cover with plastic wrap, and microwave for about 8 minutes or until almost tender. Peel sweet potatoes, and cut into ½-inch slices. Put in a medium-sized pot, cover with water, and steam for 15 minutes. While the potatoes are cooking, finely chop the onion, and sauté in olive oil. Drain potatoes. In a greased, 2-quart baking dish, spoon carrots on the bottom, then layer the sweet potatoes on top. Put sautéed onions over the potatoes. Mix the sugar into the sour cream, and spoon on top of the casserole. Sprinkle cheese over the sour cream. Bake for 20 minutes, or until cheese is melted and dish is steaming hot. For variety, add ½ cup sliced almonds over potatoes. Makes 6 to 8 servings.

Doctor's ℞: Soy not only helps to keep bones strong, it is suggested for people with cardiovascular disease. Soy will lower your LDL (low-density lipoprotein), the bad cholesterol, and raise the HDL (high-density lipoprotein), the good cholesterol. This food is also linked to lower cancer rates and is thought to lessen the symptoms of menopause.

———————

67. Julienne Vegetables with Lemon Butter

You need:

>3 medium-size carrots
>3 medium-size yellow squash
>2 medium-size zucchini
>1 cup broccoli cuts
>1 fresh red pepper
>1 stalk celery
>3 tablespoons butter
>⅓ cup fresh basil, chopped
>⅓ cup fresh thyme, chopped
>1 teaspoon lemon zest
>Salt and pepper to taste

To Make:

Julienne the vegetables into thin strips about 3 to 4 inches long and ¼ inch wide. Put celery and carrots together, and boil in water for 4 minutes until almost cooked. Drain; set aside. In a large frying pan, add butter and heat. Add ½ amount of the basil and thyme and all of the vegetables. Toss and stir until firm, then add in the rest of the herbs, lemon zest, salt and pepper. Makes 6 to 8 servings.

Chef's Comments: Don't let lack of time stop you from keeping bones strong! If you don't have time to make vegetable salads for dinner, choose from the myriad of prepackaged salads available at most supermarkets. You can also find washed baby carrots, chopped red and green cabbage, and broccoli florets that are ready to eat.

68. Lime Almond Brussels Sprouts

You need:

> 1 16-ounce package of frozen
>   brussels sprouts
> 1 tablespoon lime juice
> 2 tablespoons butter
> ½ cup slivered almonds
> Salt and pepper to taste

To make:

Preheat oven to 325 degrees. Cook brussels sprouts according to directions, drain, and spoon into a 1½-quart baking dish. Squeeze lime over brussels sprouts. Melt butter, and pour over the dish. Top with almonds and a dash of salt and pepper. Bake for 15 minutes. Makes 4 servings.

69. Mediterranean Garbanzos and Tomatoes

You need:

4 tablespoons extra virgin olive oil
1 medium red onion, chopped
3 cloves garlic, minced
2 cans garbanzo beans (chickpeas),
    rinsed, drained
2 ripe tomatoes, chopped
1 cucumber, thinly sliced
⅓ cup fresh basil, shredded
½ cup Parmesan cheese, shredded
¼ cup balsamic vinegar
1 teaspoon sugar
¼ teaspoon crushed red pepper
    flakes

To make:

Heat 2 tablespoons of the oil in large skillet. Add onion and garlic, then cook 5 minutes while stirring. Add garbanzo beans to skillet, cook and stir 5 minutes until heated. Spoon onto serving platter. Top beans with tomatoes, cucumber slices, and basil. Drizzle with a dressing made from 2 tablespoons olive oil, ¼ cup balsamic vinegar, 1 teaspoon sugar, and red pepper flakes. Serve warm or at room temperature on a bed of romaine or favorite lettuce.

Variations:

- Substitute soybeans for garbanzo beans. Soybeans are an important part of your bone-boosting plan. Dried soybeans can be purchased at most health food stores. Be sure to allow 3 to 4 hours cooking time before using in any recipe. (See page 260.)

70. New Potatoes, Tomatoes, and Kale

You need:

> 12 small new potatoes
> 1 tablespoon butter
> ½ tablespoon extra light olive oil
> 3 small garlic cloves, minced
> 4 cups (packed) kale, washed, drained
> 2 tomatoes, chopped
> Salt and pepper, to taste
> ½ cup Parmesan cheese, grated

To make:

In a medium saucepan, cover potatoes by ½ inch with salt water and bring to a boil; simmer 12 to 15 minutes. Drain potatoes; cool, then cut into halves. In a heavy skillet, melt butter and oil over moderate heat. Sauté potatoes, cut sides down, until golden or about 4 to 5 minutes. Loosen potatoes from bottom of skillet using a metal spatula, and place in a greased dish. Add garlic to skillet and cook, stirring until garlic is pale in color. Add kale and cook until wilted (about 5 minutes). During the last minute, mix chopped tomato with remaining ingredients in the skillet. Season with salt and pepper to taste. Spoon this mixture over sauted potatoes, and sprinkle with Parmesan cheese. Broil until bubbly, then serve. Makes 4 to 6 servings.

Variations:

- Substitute spinach for kale.
- Sprinkle with reduced-fat cheese of your choice such as cheddar, Jack, Gorgonzola, mozzarella, or Romano.
- Substitute a 16-ounce can of fresh cut tomatoes drained (or spicy varieties such as basil and garlic, or garlic and onion).

71. One Potato, Two Potato, Three Potato, and More!

You need:

>2 large sweet potatoes
>2 large white potatoes
>4 to 6 red potatoes
>2 teaspoons extra light olive oil
>½ teaspoon Salt Free Garlic and
>   Herb Seasoning (McCormick)
>½ teaspoon white pepper
>1 teaspoon curry powder
>¼ teaspoon nutmeg

To make:

Preheat oven to 425 degrees. Peel sweet potatoes and white potatoes, cutting each into fourths. Place potatoes in a bowl, and pour olive oil over the cut potatoes. Cut the unpeeled red potatoes into 4 sections, and add to the other potatoes. Toss to distribute the olive oil. In a bowl, combine the spices, and sprinkle them over the potatoes, coating evenly. Place potatoes on a greased baking sheet in a single layer, cut side up, and bake for 20 to 25 minutes or until tender. Makes 6 servings.

Doctor's ℞: Some studies reveal that caffeine may rob you of calcium. If you drink coffee, be sure to add extra calcium supplementation to your diet or *drink 1 cup of milk per cup of coffee* to help offset this negative calcium balance.

---

72. Orange Baked Squash

You need:

> 2 acorn squash
> Dash salt and pepper
> 2 tablespoons butter, melted
> ¼ cup calcium-fortified orange
>   juice
> ½ cup chives
> 1 tablespoon orange zest (page 278)
> 1 tablespoon sliced almonds

To make:

Preheat oven to 400 degrees. Clean acorn squash, take out seeds, then cut squash into ½-inch rings, leaving skin intact. Sprinkle with salt and pepper, then place rings in 2-quart greased baking dish. Pour melted butter and orange juice over rings, and top with chives and grated orange zest. Cover with foil, and bake for 55 to 60 minutes or until tender. Spoon sauce over rings, top with almonds, and serve. Makes 4 servings.

Chef's Comments: Marinades help foods absorb flavors, and the longer you marinate food, including tofu, the stronger the flavor will be. If you make more marinade than you need for one recipe, keep unused marinade refrigerated for up to one week in an airtight container.

73. Spinach Cheddar Frittata

You need:

> 3 leeks, thinly sliced (white part)
> 1 red pepper, cut into ¼-inch strips
> Dash garlic powder
> 2 tablespoons olive oil
> 3 cups fresh spinach, cut up
> ½ teaspoon curry powder
> ½ teaspoon onion powder
> ½ teaspoon salt
> ½ teaspoon pepper
> 1 tablespoon fresh basil, chopped
> 1 cup reduced-fat sharp cheddar
> cheese
> 12 ounces egg substitute (or 4 eggs
> and 2 egg whites)
> 2 tomatoes, thinly sliced

To make:

Preheat oven to 350 degrees. In a large sauce pan on medium-high heat, sauté sliced leeks, peppers, and garlic powder in olive oil for several minutes. Add spinach, and sauté until limp. Add curry powder, onion powder, salt and pepper, and fresh basil. Stir in cheese and egg substitute (or eggs). Pour one-half of the mixture into a 3- to 4-quart baking dish coated with nonstick spray. Top with tomatoes, then pour the rest of the spinach mixture over the tomatoes. Bake for 15 to 20 minutes, or until fairly firm in the center. Cool slightly, and cut into squares. Makes 8 servings.

Soy

74. Broccoli, Potato, and Two Cheeses

You need:

>3 pounds white potatoes
>Dash and ½ teaspoon salt
>½ teaspoon pepper
>¼ teaspoon nutmeg
>½ cup fat-free or low-fat calcium-
> fortified milk
>4 ounces silken tofu
>½ cup fat-free or low-fat ricotta
> cheese
>2 cups fresh broccoli florets,
> cooked
>⅔ cup grated Colby cheese

To make:

Preheat oven to 375 degrees. Peel potatoes, and chop into bite-size pieces. In a medium-sized pot, cover potatoes with water, add dash of salt, and boil potatoes for about 20 minutes, or until tender. Drain potatoes. In a large bowl combine potatoes, ½ teaspoon salt, pepper, and nutmeg; set aside. In a blender, combine milk, tofu, and ricotta. Blend until smooth. Using a mixer on low speed, slowly whip this cheese mixture into potatoes. Mix until combined but potatoes are still chunky. In a 4-quart baking dish sprayed with nonstick spray, put half of potatoes on the bottom, and top with all of the broccoli and half of the Colby cheese. Add another layer of potatoes, and top with the remaining half of the Colby cheese. Bake for 30 minutes. Makes 6 to 8 servings.

75. Fruity Tofu Smoothie

You need:

> ½ cup soft tofu or silken tofu
> (thickened with calcium
> sulfate)
> ½ cup fat-free plain yogurt
> ½ cup fat-free or low-fat calcium-
> enriched milk
> 1 cup fresh strawberries
> 1 teaspoon vanilla extract (or other
> flavored extract)
> Sugar or honey (sweeten to taste)

To make:

Put all ingredients in blender and process until creamy. Makes 1 serving. This bone-boosting drink is also high in protein and makes an excellent start to anyone's day, or for a quick afternoon boost.

Variations:

- Substitute seasonal fruit such as blueberries, raspberries, peaches, pineapple, or dates.
- Use frozen fruit for a thicker shake.
- Blend with two frozen milk cubes (see page 289) to make the drink thicker and even richer in calcium.

76. Meatless Chili Crumble

You need:

1 large onion, chopped
1 large bell pepper, chopped
2 tablespoons olive oil
1 12-ounce package of prebrowned, all-vegetable protein crumbles, frozen
2 cups water or low-sodium broth
4 16-ounce cans fresh-cut canned tomatoes, garlic and onion (or favorite flavor)
2 15-ounce cans dark kidney beans, drained
2 cups soybeans, cooked, drained (optional)
½ teaspoon Salt Free Garlic and Herb Seasoning (McCormick)
½ teaspoon onion powder
1 teaspoon chilli powder
½ teaspoon red pepper
1 tablespoon Worcestershire sauce
Salt and pepper, to taste
1 4-ounce can chilies (optional)
2 tablespoons fresh cilantro
3 cups brown rice, cooked according to directions (optional)
½ cup fat-free or light sour cream (optional)
½ cup low-fat sharp cheddar cheese (optional)

To make:

In a large soup pot, sauté chopped onion and pepper in olive oil on medium-high heat for 3 to 4 minutes. Add protein crumbles, and cook 4 minutes longer. Add water or broth, tomatoes, drained kidney beans, soybeans, spices,

Worcestershire sauce, and chilies. Adjust spices, then add salt and pepper to taste. Cover and cook on low for 2 hours to thicken sauce. Add cilantro just before serving, then serve over brown rice. Top each bowl of Chili Crumble with a dollop of sour cream and a sprinkle of cheese. Makes 12 servings. Recipe can be frozen and served at a later date.

Doctor's ℞: Cut back on salt to keep your bones strong. Studies show that sodium restriction reduces calcium excretion and may reduce bone loss and hip fractures.

---

77. Mexican Tempeh over Almond Rice

You need:

2 cups brown rice
1 large onion, finely chopped
2 packages tempeh, cut into 1-inch cubes
2 tablespoons olive oil
4 zucchini, cut into ¼-inch slices
1 green bell pepper, chopped
1 red pepper, chopped
1 jalapeño, finely chopped
2 cups corn, frozen
1 tablespoon lime juice
1 15-ounce can of black beans, rinsed, drained
1 32-ounce can crushed tomatoes
1 tablespoon cilantro
½ cup slivered almonds
½ cup shredded sharp cheddar cheese (optional)

To make:

Cook rice according to package directions. While rice is cooking, cut up onion and tempeh, then using a large heavy pot, sauté for 5 minutes in 2 tablespoons olive oil until tempeh is light brown. Cut up zucchini, green bell pepper, red pepper, and jalapeño, and add to the onion-tempeh mixture. Add corn, lime juice, black beans, and tomatoes. Cook over medium heat for 40 minutes. Add cilantro, and cook for an additional 5 minutes. Add almonds to the brown rice, and serve with the Mexican tempeh sauce. Top with grated cheddar cheese. Makes 4 to 6 servings.

Chef's Comments: Be sure to use low-fat, fat-free, or skim milk for drinking and in recipes. Two percent milk contains nearly 5 grams of fat, while skim or fat-free milk contains less than 1 gram of fat with 86 calories per cup.

78. Soybeans

You need:

>   2 cups dried soybeans
>   8 cups water
>   ⅓ cup vegetable oil
>   1 teaspoon salt

To make:

In a heavy soup pot, combine soybeans and water, cover, and soak over night. Before cooking, rinse beans carefully, then put back in soup pot with 8 cups of water. Add vegetable oil and salt. Simmer for 3 to 4 hours, or until desired tenderness. Makes 10 servings.

Variations:

*   Use soybeans in chili, bean dips, soups, vegetable casseroles, or any recipe that calls for dried beans.

79. Soybean Bake

You need:

> 1 large onion, chopped
> 1 tablespoon extra light olive oil
> Dash garlic powder
> Dash onion powder
> 2 cups soybeans, cooked (see page 260)
> 1 28-ounce can vegetarian baked beans, drained
> 4 tablespoons catsup
> 4 tablespoons brown sugar
> 2 tablespoons black strap molasses (optional)
> 3 tablespoons mustard
> 1 teaspoon black pepper

To make:

Preheat oven to 350 degrees. Using a large skillet, sauté chopped onion in olive oil on medium-high heat until soft; add garlic and onion powder, and stir. In a large bowl, pour in soybeans, along with the vegetarian beans; gently stir. Add cooked onions, catsup, brown sugar, black strap molasses, mustard, pepper, and spices, adjusting amounts to taste. Pour into greased 2-quart baking dish. Bake uncovered for 35 minutes until hot and bubbling. Serves 10 to 12.

Variations:

- Substitute lima beans, black beans, or kidney beans for part of the vegetarian beans.
- Add red and green peppers chunks. Be sure to sauté with onion before adding to beans.

80. Three-Cheese Spinach and Tofu Lasagna

You need:

2 cups béchamel sauce (page 208)
16 ounce whole wheat lasagna
  noodles
1 large onion, chopped
½ pound mushrooms, sliced
2 tablespoons olive oil
2 16-ounce bags fresh spinach
¼ cup fresh basil
2 tablespoons oregano (or 1
  teaspoon dried oregano)
Dash plus ¼ teaspoon salt
½ teaspoon pepper
¼ teaspoon nutmeg
½ teaspoon garlic powder
1 32-ounce container fat-free or
  low-fat ricotta cheese
8 ounces silken tofu
½ teaspoon Salt Free Garlic and
  Herb Seasoning (McCormick)
1 cup natural Parmesan cheese,
  grated
1 cups light mozzarella cheese,
  grated

To make:

Preheat oven to 350 degrees. Boil noodles according to directions and drain; set aside. In a medium sauce pan, sauté chopped onion and sliced mushrooms in olive oil for 5 to 6 minutes, or until onion pieces are clear. Steam cleaned spinach in a medium-size pot on the stove top with ½ cup water until wilted; drain, and pat dry. Stir onions, mushrooms, basil, and oregano into spinach, then add salt, pepper, nutmeg, and garlic. In the blender or food processor, blend ricotta cheese and tofu. Add dash of salt and Salt Free Garlic and Herb Seasoning. Spread 2 tablespoons of the ricotta cheese-tofu mixture over the bottom of a 3- to 4-quart baking dish sprayed with nonstick spray, then make three layers in this order: ⅓ cup noodles, ⅓ cup spinach mixture, ⅓ cup ricotta cheese-tofu mixture, ⅓ cup Parmesan cheese, and ⅓ cup mozzarella cheese. Spray foil with nonstick spray on one side, and place that side down to cover lasagna. The nonstick spray will help keep the cheese from sticking. Bake for 1 hour or until lasagna is bubbly. Let stand for 30 minutes before serving. Makes 8 to 10 servings.

81. Sweet Tomato Cream

You need:

> 1 large onion, chopped
> 1 red pepper, cut into ¼-inch slices
> 2 tablespoons extra light olive oil
> ½ teaspoon onion powder
> ½ teaspoon Salt Free Garlic and
>   Herb Seasoning (McCormick)
> ½ teaspoon pepper
> Salt to taste
> 1 tablespoon sugar
> 2 14.5-ounce cans tomatoes, diced
>   or chopped
> 1 6-ounce can tomato paste
> ¾ cup water
> ½ cup silken tofu
> 3 bay leaves
> ½ cup fresh basil and oregano,
>   combined (if you do not have fresh,
>   use ¼ cup combined)
> ½ cup Parmesan cheese, grated

To make:

In a large skillet, sauté onion and red pepper in olive oil until tender on medium-high heat. Add onion powder, Salt Free Garlic and Herb Seasoning, and pepper to skillet, stirring until blended. Salt to taste. While stirring, add sugar, 1 can chopped tomatoes, tomato paste, and water. In a blender, pour the other can of chopped tomatoes and silken tofu; blend until smooth. Pour mixture into the skillet with sauce, and continue to stir over medium heat. Add bay leaves and combined oregano and basil. Simmer for 15 minutes, then serve hot over cooked pasta with favorite roasted vegetables. Sprinkle natural Parmesan on top. Makes 6 servings.

Doctor's ℞: Eighty percent of American women do not get adequate amounts of calcium in their diet. Factors such as extreme weight loss can cause bone density to plummet to very low levels, and in some cases, it never recovers. Low calcium intake during adolescence can also limit peak bone density, as can certain medications and a host of risk factors. Be sure to use the many bone-boosting foods in this guide to ensure strong bones all your life.

———————

82. Wild Rice and Broccoli Cream

You need:

> 1 10-ounce package long grain wild rice
> 1 small onion, chopped
> 1 cup celery, chopped
> 1 tablespoon margarine
> 1 16-ounce package frozen broccoli,
> chopped
> 2 cups béchamel sauce (page 208)
> 4 ounces soft tofu
> 1 tablespoon lemon juice
> ½ cup natural Parmesan cheese,
> shredded
> 4 ounces light cream cheese
> Salt and pepper to taste

To make:

Preheat oven to 375 degrees. Cook the wild rice according to directions; set aside. Sauté chopped onion and celery in margarine to soften. Add to the cooked rice, and put the rice mixture into a lightly greased 2-quart baking dish. Cook the broccoli according to directions. Make the béchamel sauce while the broccoli is cooking. Add the tofu, lemon juice, half of the Parmesan cheese, and the cream cheese to the béchamel sauce and stir until blended. Add salt and pepper to taste. Put the broccoli over the rice and top with the sauce. Top the sauce with the remaining Parmesan cheese. Bake for 30 minutes. Makes 6 to 8 servings.

Variations:

- Add water chestnuts when you put the celery and onions in the rice.
- Try spinach instead of broccoli.

Chef's Comments: Try to use low-sodium versions of products such as soy sauce, soups, vegetable juices, and bottled marinades in bone-boosting recipes.

———————

Desserts
83. Fresh Fruit Tartlet

You need:

Tartlet and filling

> ½ cup fat-free or light cream cheese
> ½ cup soft tofu
> 1 teaspoon vanilla
> ½ cup powdered sugar (or to taste)
> 1 package frozen prepared tartlets (in
>   frozen food section near fruit)

Topping

> ¼ cup fat-free or low-fat sour cream
> ½ teaspoon orange zest (see page 278)
> 1 tablespoon powdered sugar (or to taste)
> 1 cup of seasonal fruit, such as:
>   strawberries, sliced
>   kiwi, sliced
>   bananas, sliced and dipped in citrus juice
>   orange segments
>   apricots, sliced
>   raspberries
>   blueberries

To make:

In a small bowl, make the filling by blending the cream cheese, tofu, vanilla, and powdered sugar to taste. If you are not familiar with the flavor of tofu, you may want to add a little more powdered sugar to sweeten. In a separate bowl, prepare the topping by mixing sour cream, orange zest, and 1 tablespoon powdered sugar (or to taste). Prepare fruit, and set aside. Fill each tartlet ¾ full of filling, then put 1 teaspoon of sour cream topping over filling; add fruit for decoration. Refrigerate until time of serving. Makes 8 to 12 servings.

84. Gourmet Fruit with Vanilla Bean Syrup

You need:

> 2 cups water
> 1 cup sugar
> 1 vanilla bean (split)
> ⅓ cup orange liqueur
> Use a combination of seasonal fruit
> to equal 6 cups, such as:
> cantaloupe balls
> honeydew balls
> watermelon balls
> blueberries
> green or red grapes
> cherries
> fresh pineapple, cored and cut
> into rings
> strawberries, with tops cut off
> bananas, dipped in citrus juice
> oranges, peeled and cut in
> segments
> kiwi, peeled, sliced

To make:

In a medium saucepan, combine water, sugar, and the vanilla bean that has been split lengthwise. (By splitting the bean lengthwise you will release the seeds and enhance the flavor.) Boil over moderately high heat for 5 to 10 minutes, stirring down the sugar crystals that form along the side of the pan and until slightly thickened. Cool the syrup, then add the orange liqueur. While the vanilla syrup is chilling, prepare fruit of choice. Layer fruit in a large (10-cup) clear glass bowl or compote in a decorative manner. For example, start with a layer of pineapple rings on the bottom, add strawberries (layering decoratively around the edges of the bowl or compote), then bananas, orange segments, more pineapple and strawberries, honeydew, red grapes, bananas, and blueberries. Top the layers of fruit with kiwi and a few strawberries for decoration. This can also be done in individual parfait glasses. When the syrup is cooled, pour over the fruit, and let marinate for 6 to 8 hours. Makes 8 servings.

85. Guava Bread Pudding

You need:

> 1 loaf calcium-fortified bread
> 4 cups fat-free or low-fat calcium-
>   fortified milk
> 1 tablespoon vanilla
> 1 cup sugar
> ¼ cup butter
> 1 10-ounce jar guava jelly (or 1 can
>   guava paste)

To make:

Preheat oven to 325 degrees. Crumble the entire loaf of bread, and put in a greased 4-quart baking dish. Pour the milk and vanilla over this, and soak for 1 hour in the refrigerator. Mix in the sugar and butter. Spoon guava jelly (or guava paste slices) over bread mixture; bake uncovered for 45 minutes. The sugar forms a delicate, crispy outer layer with a moist bread pudding. This can be served with prepared whipped topping (fat-free is good). Makes 10 to 12 servings.

Variations:

- Use light or low-fat margarine instead of butter to cut fat calories.
- Use your favorite all-fruit preserves instead of guava.

86. Jewel's Apple Crumble

You need:

> 1 cup flour
> ¼ teaspoon nutmeg
> ½ teaspoon cinnamon
> ¼ teaspoon salt
> 1 cup brown sugar, packed
> ½ cup butter
> 1 teaspoon lemon rind (zest) (page 278)
> 1 tablespoon lemon juice
> 6 medium apples, peeled, cored, sliced
> ½ cup walnuts, chopped

To make:

Preheat oven to 350 degrees. Sift flour, spices, and salt together in a medium bowl. Add ¾ cup brown sugar (reserving ¼ cup brown sugar for topping), then cut softened butter into the dry mixture. Sprinkle ⅓ of the crumb mixture into a 1½-quart baking dish; set aside. Grate the lemon in a small bowl to get 1 tablespoon lemon zest; set aside. In a medium bowl, combine peeled-and-sliced apples and chopped walnuts with lemon juice and zest. Spoon the apple mixture over the small amount of crumb mixture in the baking dish, then top with the remaining crumb mixture. Sprinkle the reserved ¼ cup brown sugar over the casserole. Cover with foil, and bake for 30 minutes. Remove the foil, and cook an additional 20 minutes. Serve with Light and Elegant Whipped Topping (page 274). Makes 6 to 8 servings.

Variations:

- Use ¼ cup soy flour in place of regular flour.

Doctor's ℞: There are many available tests your doctor can use to test your bone density. These are quick, easy, and do not cause any discomfort. Most health insurers will pay for this test if you have a fracture, are postmenopausal, if you are not taking estrogen at menopause, or if you are taking medications which can cause bone thinning. Medicare will also pay for a bone density test for women over age 65.

———————

87. Layered Ambrosia

You need:

> 1 cup fresh coconut, grated (if not available, use packaged sweet coconut)
> 15 fresh oranges
> 3 tablespoons sugar
> ½ cup cherries (optional)
> ½ cup bananas, sliced (optional)
> ½ cup pecans, chopped (optional)

To make:

On a hard surface outside, put coconut on a dishtowel or several paper towels to catch milk that is released when cracked. Place a screwdriver into coconut, and hit with a hammer to crack coconut in two halves. With a knife, carefully pull chunks of coconut meat away from the shell and grate, freezing any excess for later use. Peel the oranges, cutting the skin away to the pulp so that no skin is left. Separate into segments, and place ⅓ of the oranges in the bottom of a medium-size bowl or compote. Sprinkle ⅓ of the coconut and 1 tablespoon of sugar over the oranges; layer another ⅓ of oranges, coconut, and sugar until all are used. If you desire, add additional fruit or nuts in each layer. Makes 8 servings.

Chef's Comments: Soybeans surpass all other plant-based foods in the amount of protein they can deliver to the body. If you are cooking dried soybeans, make enough for several meals. Freeze extra beans and broth in zippered freezer bags to use in future recipes.

———————

88. Light and Elegant Whipped Topping

You need:

> 1 teaspoon gelatin
> 2 teaspoons cold water
> 3 tablespoons boiling water
> ½ cup ice water
> ½ cup nonfat dry milk
> 3 tablespoons sugar
> 3 tablespoons vegetable oil
> 1 teaspoon citrus zest (lemon, lime
>   or orange) (page 278)

To make:

Chill a medium-size bowl to whip nonfat dry milk. Using small bowl, soften gelatin in cold water. Stir, then add boiling water. Continue to stir until water becomes tepid (neither cool nor hot to touch). Pour ice water and nonfat dry milk into the chilled bowl, beating until stiff. Add sugar, oil, and gelatin mixture. Beat briefly, then stir in citrus zest. Freeze immediately for 15 minutes and serve. Use with any dish that calls for whipped cream or whipped topping. Makes 4 servings.

89. Pumpkin Flan

You need:

> 1⅓ cups sugar
> 2¼ cups fat-free or low-fat calcium
>   fortified milk
> 6 ounces egg substitute (or 3 large
>   eggs)
> 3 egg whites
> 1½ cups pumpkin, canned
> 1 teaspoon pumpkin pie spice
> ½ teaspoon cinnamon
> ½ teaspoon ginger
> 1 teaspoon vanilla extract
> 3 tablespoons pecans, chopped

To make:

Preheat oven to 350 degrees. Spoon ½ cup sugar into a 9×13-inch metal baking dish. Using an oven mitt, carefully hold pan over medium heat until the sugar melts and turns golden in color. Shake occasionally to keep sugar from burning. Heat milk and remaining sugar, stirring until hot. Beat egg substitute, egg whites, pumpkin, and spices at low speed with an electric mixer until thoroughly blended. Slowly add hot milk mixture to this, beating on medium-low speed. Pour mixture over the golden brown sugar in baking dish. Place baking dish in a larger roasting pan that has been filled with 1-inch water. Bake for 1 hour. Test with a clean knife inserted in center of flan to see if it is done. If the knife comes out clean, take the flan out and cool on a wire rack. Bake pecans in a small cakepan in the 350-degree oven for 5 minutes or until brown. Chill the flan for at least 6 hours, then gently loosen the edges of the flan with a spatula and invert on a serving plate; top with chopped pecans and a spoon of favorite whipped cream or Light and Elegant Whipped Topping (page 274). Makes 6 to 8 servings.

90. White Chocolate Mousse

You need:

> 8 ounces white chocolate, cut into
>   pieces
> ½ cup whipping cream (half and
>   half is okay, but not quite as thick)
> ½ cup silken tofu
> 1 tablespoon butter
> 1 tablespoon sugar
> 2 tablespoons rum
> 1 teaspoon orange zest (optional)
> ½ cup fresh fruit (sliced
>   strawberries, raspberries,
>   kiwi, or blueberries)

To make:

Melt the white chocolate over a medium-size double boiler. Or put the chocolate in a small saucepan, and place this in a larger pot filled with 1-inch water. Once this is melted, add the tofu, whipping cream, butter, and sugar. Continue to cook until all ingredients are combined. Take this off the unit, and continue stirring with wooden spoon until completely blended. Add rum, and allow mixture to cool. Stir in orange rind, then spoon into individual serving dishes. Cool in refrigerator. Top with fresh fruit slices when ready to serve. Makes 4 servings.

Quick and Easy Kids' Food
91. Crazy Kids' Mix

You need:

- ½ cup peanuts
- 4 ounces sunflower seeds
- ½ cup soy nuts
- 6 ounces Tropical Fruit Mix
  (Delmonte)
- 3½ ounces dried cherries
- ¼ cup raisins
- 4 ounces chocolate raisins
- 3½ ounces yogurt raisins
- ¼ cup dates, chopped
- ½ cup M&M's
- ¼ cup chocolate chips

To make:

In a medium-size bowl, combine any assortment of the above ingredients that your child enjoys eating. Try to include as many of the bone-boosting foods as possible, and store in an airtight container. Put in small bags for lunch boxes or serve for afterschool snacks. Number of servings depends on amount used.

Doctor's ℞: Manganese is an important bone booster. You can ensure a diet high in manganese by eating whole grain products, beans and nuts, sweet potatoes and eggs, as well as leafy green vegetables.

———————————

92. Orangeman Cupcakes

You need:

> 2⅔ cups flour
> 4 teaspoons baking powder
> ½ teaspoon salt
> 1½ cups sugar
> ⅓ cup fat-free or low-fat calcium-
>   fortified milk
> ⅔ cup orange juice
> 4 ounces egg substitute (or 2 eggs)
> ⅓ cup Lighter Bake (or 1 stick
>   butter)

Icing:

> ¼ tablespoons orange juice
> 2 cups confectioners sugar
> 1 tablespoon orange rind (zest)
> Dash salt

To make:

Preheat oven to 400 degrees. Prepare pan with muffin paper cups. In a large mixing bowl, combine flour, baking powder, salt, and sugar. Add milk, orange juice, eggs, and ⅓ cup Lighter Bake (or softened butter). Blend until ingredients are mixed. Pour into muffin paper cups, filling about ¾ full. Bake for approximately 20 minutes. Using a sharp knife, test the center of the cupcakes. If the knife does not come out clean, cook 5 minutes longer. Prepare icing in a medium-size bowl, and stir until blended. Ice cupcakes when cool. Makes 12 to 16 cupcakes.

Chef's Comments: To make citrus zest: Using clean citrus, take a grater and place over a plate. Rub fruit up and down on medium grate until desired "zest" is produced. Do not grate the pectin—just the outer skin of the fruit. You can purchase a "zester" at most kitchen shops that are easy to use and safe.

Picky Parties—A Bone-Boosting Party Snack for Each Day of the Week

93. Picky Party 1—Sweet Treat

You need:

> ½ cup creamy peanut butter
> 1 tablespoon honey
> Your choice of fruit or veggies,
>   such as:
>   apple slices
>   banana chunks
>   celery sticks
>   dates
>   pear slices
> 4 slices calcium-enriched bread

Face decorations:

- chopped dates
- raisins
- nuts (almonds, sunflower seeds, walnuts, pecans, peanuts, or soy nuts)

To make:

Let your child measure the peanut butter, then scoop it into a small bowl. Measure the honey, and mix into the peanut butter. Spread the peanut butter–honey mixture onto the bread, then let your child use the assorted fruit, veggies, and nuts to decorate the slice of bread, making a funny face to eat. Makes 4 servings.

94. Picky Party 2—Nasty Nachos

You need (per person):

> 10 tortilla chips
> ¼ cup low-fat grated cheese
> ¼ cup fresh tomato salsa

To make:

On a baking sheet, place tortilla chips in a single layer, allowing about 10 chips per child. Top the chips with the grated cheese. Broil until the cheese begins to melt. Cool slightly, and serve with the fresh tomato salsa or the salsa of your choice.

95. Picky Party 3—Beans in a Bun

You need (per person):

> 1 hot dog or hamburger bun
> 1 slice low-fat cheese (or substitute
>   American or jalapeño Jack
>   fat-free soy cheese)
> 2 tablespoons Soybean Bake,
>   prepared (see page 261)

To make:

Split bun in half, and put 2 tablespoons soybean bake on one side. Top with a slice of cheese. Broil until cheese is melted. Cool slightly and serve.

Variation:

- Top cheese with a large slice of Vidalia onion or tomato before broiling.

96. Picky Party 4—Veg-Out Bagel

You need:

> 1 bagel per person
> 4 ounces fat-free or low-fat cream
>   cheese
> ¼ cup red, green, or yellow
>   peppers, chopped
> ¼ cup green onions, chopped
> ¼ cup carrots, finely chopped

To make:

Split bagel in half. Blend cream cheese and vegetables together in a small bowl. Spread on bagel and serve. Refrigerate remaining spread. The cream cheese will make 4 to 6 servings.

Variation:

- In place of vegetables, try cranberries and orange juice. In a blender, put 1 tablespoon cranberries, a 1-inch square of orange peel, 1 tablespoon orange juice, and cream cheese. Blend, scraping down the sides of the blender jar, and continue until cranberries are totally blended. Makes 4 to 6 servings.

Doctor's ℞: If you cannot use dairy products, try any of the following nondairy foods. Each one contains enough calcium to equal an 8-ounce cup of milk: 5.7 ounces of dry roasted almonds, 4 cups of cauliflower, 2.5 cups of broccoli or white beans, 2 cups of rutabaga, 1 cup of Chinese cabbage or turnip greens, or ½ cup of calcium-set tofu.

97. Picky Party 5—Kiddie Quesadillas

You need (per person):

> 1 tortilla
> 1 slice fat-free or low-fat cheese
> 1 teaspoon margarine

To make:

Lay the cheese on one half of the tortilla. Fold the tortilla over. Heat a skillet, and put the margarine in the pan. Put the tortilla on the margarine, lightly brown one side then the other. Serve with favorite fruit slices.

Variation:

• Use salsa (page 166) as a dip for the tortilla.

Chef's Comments: To wilt spinach, put fresh spinach in a large microwave-proof bowl with ½ cup water. Cover and cook for 10 minutes on high. Drain spinach thoroughly, then pat dry with a paper towel before using in recipes.

98. Picky Party 6—Soft and Squeezy Tacos

You need (per person):

> 1 tortilla
> ¼ cup fat-free or low-fat cheese,
>   grated
> 1 tablespoon tomato, chopped
> 1 tablespoon fat-free or low-fat
>   sour cream

To make:

Lay the tortilla on a paper towel, and place on a microwave-proof plate. Sprinkle cheese down the center of the tortilla, then top with tomato and sour cream. Roll tortilla; with seam side down, wrap in the paper towel, and microwave for 1 minute. Cool slightly and serve.

Variations:

- Add chopped green onions over tomatoes.
- Add a leaf of spinach and microwave for 1½ minutes.

99. Picky Party 7—Veg-Out Dip

You need:

> Assorted fresh vegetables, cut into
> kid-size pieces (broccoli
> florets, carrot and celery sticks,
> slices of yellow squash,
> zucchini, and red, green, and
> yellow peppers)

To make:

Make Spicy Salmon Dip (page 175), Southwestern Bean
and Cheese Dip (page 173), or Parmesan Spinach Dip (page
171), and let children use fresh vegetables for dipping. Eliminate horseradish or any spices from the recipe that may be
unappealing to young children. Makes 8 servings.

100. Simon's Brown Bread Yogurt

You need:

>   ½ gallon calcium-fortified frozen
>   vanilla yogurt
>   2 cups calcium-fortified brown
>   bread crumbs (about 5 to 6
>   slices, crumbled in blender)
>   ¼ cup sugar
>   Fat-free whipped topping (see page
>   274)

To make:

Preheat oven to 350 degrees. Take yogurt out of freezer, and let soften while preparing bread crumbs. In a large bowl, mix bread crumbs with sugar until coated. On an air-bake cookie sheet, spread out crumbs. Bake crumbs for 25 minutes, stirring at intervals of 10 minutes until done. Crumbs will be a medium brown when completely cooked. If they are pale, continue cooking for 5 minutes. Let the crumbs cool. Blend the softened yogurt and baked crumbs in a large bowl. Cover with foil, and refreeze for several hours or until hardened. Serve with fat-free whipped topping. Serves 10.

Variations:

- Purchase whole wheat bread that is high in calcium (at least 100 to 140 mg per slice).
- Vary your flavors of yogurt, or use fat-free or light ice cream.
- Top with fresh fruit such as sliced apricots, strawberries, and peaches.
- Put crumbs in fat-free or low-fat calcium-fortified yogurt for a quick breakfast.
- Using the crumbs, create your own granola, adding dried apricots, apples, raisins, or dates.

101. Spicy Hummus

You need:

¼ cup tahini (sesame seed paste)
    or 3 tablespoons creamy
    peanut butter
3 tablespoons lemon juice
3 tablespoons nonfat dry milk
3 garlic cloves, minced
2 cans garbanzo beans and liquid
    (if using cooked dried beans—
    2½ cups cooked with ¼ cup
    broth)
1 teaspoon ground cumin
½ teaspoon crushed red pepper
Extra water, if needed, for
    blending
Salt to taste

To make:

Using your food processor, puree tahini (or peanut butter),
lemon juice, milk, and garlic. Add garbanzo beans and liquid
(½ cup at a time). When all ingredients are thoroughly
blended, stir in cumin and red pepper; add salt to taste.
Keeps well in refrigerator up to 5 days.

Variations:

- Use hummus as a spread for school lunch sandwiches. Add bean sprouts, roasted vegetables, and
  shredded fresh vegetables for texture and flavor.
- Put hummus in a plastic container for school
  lunches. Add chopped vegetables or bagel slices
  for dipping.

102. Yam Ma'am (Sweet Potato Faces)

You need:

> 1 medium yam (sweet potato)
> Margarine for coating, as needed
> Assorted toppings, such as:
>> marshmallows
>> raisins
>> peanuts, almonds, walnuts, or
>>> sunflower seeds (great for
>>> ma'am's hair!)
>> dried fruit (apricots, dates, or
>>> apples, chopped)

To make:

Preheat oven to 400 degrees. Wash yam, and grease with a small amount of margarine. Puncture yam with a fork several times on each side. Place on a baking sheet, and bake for 50 to 60 minutes, depending on the size of the potato. Test the center of the potato with a fork to make sure it is soft. Let the potato cool; slice in half lengthwise, and let the children decorate with their favorite toppings. Use the fruit, nuts, or marshmallows to make the face (eyes, nose, and mouth). Use sunflower seeds for hair. You can broil briefly to set the marshmallows, then cool, and let the kids dig in. Makes 2 servings per sweet potato.

Variations:

- Brush the potato halves with margarine and sprinkle a little brown sugar and cinnamon before decorating.
- Brush each potato half with a mixture of 1 tablespoon orange juice and 1 tablespoon butter. Sprinkle with brown sugar and cinnamon before decorating.

101 Bone-Boosting Makeovers

1. If you are allergic to cow's milk, consider calcium-fortified soy milk or rice milk for cooking (1 cup = 300 mg).

2. If a recipe calls for 1 cup milk (300 mg calcium), replace this with calcium-fortified milk (1 cup = 500 mg calcium).

3. Add 2 tablespoons milk powder (400 mg calcium) to a glass of skim milk (300 mg calcium). Stir, freeze in ice cube trays, and use instead of ice cubes for a high-calcium boost to milkshakes or smoothies.

4. Substitute cabbage for lettuce in salads and boost vitamin K (½ cup cooked = 73 mcg vitamin K).

5. Use calcium-fortified soy milk or rice milk in recipes that call for milk (1 cup = 300 mg).

6. Add barley to soup for a boost of magnesium.

7. Add chopped red and green peppers to rice prior to cooking. Consider adding chopped collard or mustard greens, kale, or spinach for an even greater bone boost.

8. Increase the vitamin content of each meal by adding fresh sliced fruit (cantaloupe, oranges, kiwi, strawberries, or grapefruit) to the plate.

9. Keep single-serving (6-ounce) cans of low-sodium vegetable juice at work to boost your intake of bone-boosting vitamins and minerals.

10. Use evaporated skim milk (½ cup = 300 mg calcium) instead of half and half in your coffee or tea.

11. Whenever possible, substitute milk for water in a recipe. Milk contains 90 percent water yet is full of bone-boosting vitamins and minerals.

12. Add salmon with bones to your lunchtime salad to increase calcium intake.

13. Add chopped broccoli and red pepper to your macaroni and cheese recipe to boost calcium

and minerals. Be sure to use calcium-fortified milk, and add extra low-fat cheese, too.

14. Use fat-free or low-fat cheese in recipes that call for regular cheese.

15. Use calcium-fortified milk instead of water for hot cereals or hot chocolate.

16. For waffles, pancakes, and puddings, add 2 tablespoons of nonfat dry milk into each cup of flour.

17. Add calcium-fortified orange juice instead of water to congealed salads (1 cup = 300 mg).

18. Sprinkle salads and vegetables with Parmesan cheese (1 tablespoon = 70 mg calcium).

19. Substitute Edy's Calcium-fortified No-fat Frozen Yogurt for recipes that call for ice cream, and get 45 percent of your day's calcium requirement for just ½ cup yogurt.

20. Use fat-free cream cheese instead of peanut butter for sandwiches or bagels (2 tablespoons = 150 mg calcium).

21. Use soy granules as a filler for meatloaf or meatballs (high in isoflavones, which help to preserve bone strength).

22. To use fat-free or low-fat cheese in a recipes, first shred or grate the cheese. Toss this with a little cornstarch to coat before you try to melt it.

23. Substitute calcium-enriched plain fat-free or low-fat yogurt in recipes that call for mayonnaise in dips, dressings, and salads (1 cup plain yogurt = 400 mg calcium).

24. Include dark leafy greens such as spinach, mustard and collard greens, and kale in soups and casseroles to boost calcium and vitamins A and K.

25. Add 2 tablespoons milk powder (400 mg calcium) to a glass of soy milk. Stir, freeze in ice cube trays, and use instead of ice cubes for a high-calcium boost to milkshakes or smoothies.

26. Instead of ground beef, try Harvest Burgers

Vegetable Protein Crumbles (Green Giant) in soups and sauces. Two-thirds of a cup of crumbles has 10 percent of your daily calcium (100 mg), 30 percent of your zinc (4.5 mg), and zero fat.

27. Give children string cheese for a snack, and add 300 mg of vitamin A and 250 mg of calcium in just one snack stick.

28. If you have trouble with dairy products, consider Lactaid Lactose-Reduced Low-Fat Cottage Cheese, 1 percent. One-half cup gives you 100 mg of calcium.

29. Check your dairy case regularly for the latest reduced-fat products. Athenos now makes a reduced-fat feta cheese. One ounce gives you 300 mg of vitamin A and 80 mg of calcium.

30. A new cheese alternative, Veggie Slices, Organic Tofu (low-fat, lactose-free, and cholesterol-free) is made by Galaxy Foods. One slice provides 500 mg of vitamin A and 200 mg of calcium. It is available in American flavor and Pepper Jack, among others.

31. Tempeh has been around for centuries. It is made from soybeans that are precooked and held together with a mold-like ingredient similar to blue cheese. One-half cup of tempeh gives you a high-protein, low-fat food source that has 550 mg of vitamin A and about 80 mg of calcium. Tempeh can be sliced, baked, grilled, or fried and is available in health food stores.

32. Experiment with *tofu* in your favorite recipes to add a new source of bone-boosting nutrients that is high in soy protein and low in fat. Tofu comes in different textures and flavors, including smoked cheese, spicy, barbecue, and roast duck. You can substitute tofu for cheese (ricotta), sour cream, meat in a stir fry, yogurt, or milk.

33. Use *extra firm tofu* for slicing, dicing, pan frying, boiling, broiling, and baking. Extra firm

tofu provides the *highest protein* content of the different types of tofu. Marinate cubed extra-firm tofu in your favorite sauce. Or try it on a skewer with veggies, and grill. Substitute tofu for meat when making fajitas, or season and sauté tofu, and put in a pita with vegetables and cheese.

34. Use *firm tofu* if you need a lighter consistency. This type provides 150 mg of calcium per serving.

35. Try *soft tofu* in soups, sauces, and salads. Soft tofu provides about 150 mg of calcium per serving.

36. If you are making desserts or smoothies, *silken tofu* will be your best selection. It has a custard-like texture. Silken tofu can be mixed in the blender with cocoa, honey, and vanilla flavoring for a sweet bone-boosting drink. Or it can be added to dips like guacamole or to quick bread batters.

37. Nasoya's Vegi-Dressings contain half the calories of regular dressing, 70 percent less fat or fat-free, and are all natural soy-based products made from silken tofu. You might try Sesame Garlic, Creamy Dill, Garden Herb, Creamy Italian, or Thousand Island on your salad or use this as a tasty dip for vegetables.

38. Fat-free sour cream seems to work as well if not better than applesauce as a substitute for oil in baked recipes and gives an extra dose of calcium without added fat.

39. Yogurt cheese can be used instead of cream cheese on bagels or as a dip. Yogurt cheese will provide a higher source of calcium, and some fat-free yogurts are only 100 calories for 8 ounces and provide 350 mg of calcium. To make: Pour a 16-ounce container of plain low-fat yogurt into a colander set in a bowl to drain, and refrigerate for 24 hours. The drained yogurt will have the consistency of cream cheese. You

can add fresh basil, cilantro, chives, onions, peppers, celery, carrots, green onions, strawberries, raspberries, blueberries, dates, or nuts to make a dip, spread, or sauce.

40. *Roasted soybeans* are one of the highest food sources for phytoestrogens. You can add them to salads for an extra bone boost. To roast soybeans: Take 2 cups of cooked soybeans, strain, and dry. Sprinkle sea salt over a baking sheet, then pour soybeans over the sheet. Bake uncovered at 350 degrees for about 45 minutes or until crispy and brown. Cool the soybeans, and store in an airtight container. If they become soggy, freshen them by baking at 200 degrees for 20 to 30 minutes, or until crisp.

41. If you want the taste of a lunch meat sandwich without the meat, look in the produce section of your grocery store for the latest varieties of soy-based food products. You will find veggie hot dogs, veggie burgers, veggie bacon, veggie pepperoni, and even veggie bologna. Most are excellent sources of protein and contain calcium.

42. Try soy milk instead of regular milk in hot chocolate, or use one-half soy milk, one-half regular milk until you get used to the change in flavor.

43. Try ¼ cup soy milk and ¾ cup 1 percent milk in recipes or over cereal. Gradually increase soy, and decrease regular milk.

44. Instead of milk, use soy milk in soups to increase isoflavone content of food.

45. Soft tofu can be substituted for half of the cream cheese in cheese cake recipes.

46. *Soy flour* adds protein and improves the crust color of baked products. It can be substituted for one-fourth to one-half of the regular flour in most recipes. Because products made with soy flour brown more quickly, be sure to cut back on your total cooking time or use a slightly

lower temperature. Check frequently if unsure. Soy flour must be stored in the refrigerator or freezer as it can become rancid.

47. Try fresh spinach (two 10- to 16-ounce bags) in lasagna recipes instead of meat. Cook the spinach, then drain off liquid and pat dry before layering in recipe.

48. Powdered *soy protein isolates* can be purchased at health food stores. This bone-boosting powder is the chief component of many dairylike products such as milk, cheese, or nondairy frozen desserts. It can be added to smoothies, casseroles, and baked goods.

49. *Black soybeans* are delicious in casseroles and chili and can be purchased at most health food stores. They are available canned or as dried uncooked legumes.

50. Make your own bread crumbs with high-calcium bread. Crumble the bread in a food processor, and store in an airtight container or freeze. Add oregano or sweet basil to make Italian bread crumbs.

51. Squeeze fresh lemon, lime, or orange juice over vegetables for an added bone boost of vitamin C.

52. Sprinkle basil, parsley, oregano, or rosemary over new potatoes, then spoon fat-free sour cream over the herb for added vitamins and minerals.

53. Make ice cubes out of fresh lemonade for an added boost of vitamin C to fruit juice, tea, or mineral water.

54. Try lemon, lime, or calcium-enriched orange juice in soups and dips for zestier flavor and more bone-boosting power.

55. Toss in bone-boosting almonds, walnuts, cashews, soybeans, pumpkin seeds, sesame seeds, sunflower seeds, Brazil nuts, or peanuts to pasta, salads, rice, couscous, and other dishes.

56. Use soy milk instead of cow's milk when making mashed potatoes. Boil potatoes until tender, then drain. Mash with soy milk, salt, pepper, garlic, and your favorite cheese.

57. Keep fruits such as apples, raisins, mango, papayas, cantaloupes, apricots, guava, strawberries, oranges, tangerines, grapefruits, kiwis, bananas, raspberries, and blueberries available for a quick supper side dish or to add to salads and casseroles.

58. Consider using sweet potatoes or yams in place of white potatoes in your favorite recipes.

59. *Soy flour* can replace eggs in many recipes. Use 1 tablespoon soy flour and 1 tablespoon water to replace one egg.

60. Bake a pumpkin for a great side dish and a huge boost of vitamin A. Cut the top off the pumpkin, and scrape out the seeds. Reserve seeds to roast later. Sprinkle brown sugar into the center of the pumpkin, then add butter to taste. Cover the pumpkin with foil, and bake just like acorn squash at 400 degrees for 1 hour or until tender.

61. Roast the pumpkin seeds to get a boost in vitamin A, calcium, magnesium, phosphorus, calcium, and zinc. Coat 2 cups cleaned and dried seeds with 1 tablespoon oil and 1 teaspoon salt. Put seeds on a baking sheet in a 250-degree oven for 30 to 40 minutes or until golden, stirring occasionally.

62. Grate carrots over salads and into sandwich spreads for a boost of vitamins A and C. Add ½ cup grated carrots and 1 tablespoon fat-free mayonnaise to 1 can water-packed tuna for a bone-boosting high-protein, low-fat lunch.

63. Foods high in vitamin E are crucial for building bones. Try to include the following in daily recipes: almonds, corn oil, cod liver oil, corn oil margarine, hazelnuts, lobster, peanut butter,

safflower oil, salmon steak, and sunflower seeds.

64. Add assorted vegetables to pizza to increase bone-boosting vitamins and minerals. A few good choices are spinach, squash, zucchini, tomatoes, artichokes, onions, broccoli, and red, green, or yellow peppers. If you feel creative, try chunks of pineapple, green bell pepper, and sliced red onion for a colorful Hawaiian-style pizza.

65. Cook frozen vegetables in calcium-fortified milk for extra flavor. For variety, add bouillon and your favorite spices to vegetables and blend in a food processor, and you have made a virtually fat-free vegetable soup.

66. Try the new yogurts available such as Dannon Light. This fat-free, high-calcium food can be added to your favorite recipes in place of sour cream or milk. Dannon Light provides 35 percent of the daily requirement for calcium per 8-ounce serving.

67. Try making bone-boosting mayonnaise out of tofu. Blend the following: 1 block tofu, ⅓ cup lemon juice, ½ teaspoon onion powder, ½ teaspoon Salt Free Garlic and Herb Seasoning (McCormick), 1 teaspoon basil, and ¼ teaspoon lemon zest. Should last up to 5 days in the refrigerator.

68. Try making whipped cream out of tofu. Be sure to check the date on the tofu for freshness, and keep only as long as recommended. Blend the following: 1 cup soft tofu, 4 tablespoons oil, ¼ cup sugar, 1 teaspoon flavoring (vanilla, rum, orange, or almond), dash salt, and ½ teaspoon lime juice. Add up to 2 tablespoons fat-free calcium-fortified milk, cream, or soy milk as needed to get the desired consistency. Spoon over fresh fruit for a real bone booster.

69. Lavishly sprinkle parsley on your favorite

dishes. One-half cup of fresh parsley has 1,500 IUs of vitamin A and 40 mg of calcium.

70. Add calcium-fortified milk to scrambled eggs. Add 2 tablespoons of milk for each beaten raw egg.

71. Beta-carotene is converted to vitamin A in the body, and vitamin A is vital for strong bones. Food sources of beta-carotene should be used each day. Try to include the highest sources including apricots, asparagus, beef liver, broccoli, cantaloupe, carrots, kale, mustard greens, spinach, sweet potato, watermelon, and yellow corn.

72. Foods rich in magnesium can easily be used in most recipes. Try to include several sources of magnesium in your daily diet by using almonds, avocado, bananas, black-eyed peas, cashews, kidney beans, lima beans, oatmeal, peanut butter, pecans, shredded wheat, soy flour, soybeans, tofu, walnuts, and whole wheat flour.

73. Use pureed fruit products such as Lighter Bake to replace butter, oil, or shortening in most recipes. Lighter Bake is a tasty combo of apples and prunes and can help keep the flavor in recipes without unnecessary fat.

74. Substitute *soft tofu* for the dairy and egg ingredients in your favorite pumpkin pie recipe

75. Substitute up to ½ cup of *silken or soft tofu* for ½ cup ricotta in recipes.

76. Add chopped vegetables such as red and green peppers, broccoli, green onions, and tomatoes to fat-free calcium-fortified cottage cheese to boost vitamins A and C and calcium in your diet.

77. Pour calcium-fortified orange juice over fruit for a bone-boosting dessert or fruit salad.

78. Use cooked, chopped vegetables such as spinach, broccoli, tomatoes, and peppers to fill a baked potato. Top with shredded natural Parmesan cheese or reduced-fat cheddar cheese,

then add a dollop of fat-free sour cream for a bone-boosting quick meal.

79.   Combine soy milk and fruit (frozen strawberries, raspberries, blueberries, blackberries, or bananas) in a blender and puree for a high-energy bone-boosting drink. Sweeten to taste.

80.   Zinc is an important bone booster. Add the following foods to favorite recipes to ensure adequate zinc in your diet: seafood, eggs, meats, whole grains, wheat germ, nuts, and seeds.

81.   Tired of the same pizza toppings? Try low-fat goat cheese, fresh wilted spinach, tomatoes, and bell peppers for an innovative bone-boosting pizza topping.

82.   Papaya sounds exotic, and this fruit gives a big boost of vitamins A and C. Try to incorporate papaya into your menus when it is in season.

83.   Choose spinach over lettuce for a bone-boosting salad. Add favorite chopped vegetables, then make a tofu-based dressing using the recipe on page 196.

84.   Apricots, pineapple, papaya, melon, mango, strawberry, kiwi, banana, raspberries, blueberries, and blackberries all make great bone-boosting additions to yogurt or cottage cheese. Stir in your favorite fruits to ½ cup fat-free calcium-fortified cottage cheese for a quick afternoon snack.

85.   Try a chocolate smoothie. Use 8 ounces silken tofu, 1 small banana, ½ cup frozen raspberries, 2 teaspoons cocoa, and 4 bone-boosting milk ice cubes (page 289). Blend until smooth.

86.   When you steam your veggies, save the broth. Freeze this in ice cube trays, then pop out the cubes, and store in a zippered freezer bag. Take out the amount needed when your recipe calls for instant low-sodium vegetable broth.

87.   When making guacamole, give it a new bone-

boosting twist. Add ½ cup pureed soybeans, ½ cup pureed chickpeas, or ½ cup fat-free ricotta cheese.

88. Popeye was right to eat his spinach! Spinach and brussels sprouts can boost your intake of vitamins A, C, and K, calcium, magnesium and phosphorus, and keep bones strong.

89. To preserve bone-boosting nutrients, avoid overcooking vegetables. Vegetables should be cooked until "crisp tender," not soggy. If unsure, cut your cooking time in half, and test the vegetables. If too crisp, cook for a minute or two until you reach the right texture.

90. Be sure to use plenty of foods rich in vitamin C as you plan your menu each day, including broccoli, cabbage, carambola or star fruit, citrus fruits, green peppers, mangoes, papayas, passion fruit, potatoes, strawberries, and tomatoes.

91. Kohlrabi, also called cabbage turnip, is very high in vitamin C. It can be used as a cabbage. Or you can sauté kohlrabi in vegetable broth, drain, and top with cheddar cheese.

92. It's very easy to get ample calcium in your diet through food, if you compare the calcium content in foods you eat each day. For example, 1 cup of plain nonfat yogurt has 400 mg of calcium, 8 ounces of calcium-fortified orange juice has 300 mg, and 8 ounces of Calcimilk (lactose-reduced with added calcium and 1 percent fat) has 500 mg. If you ate these three foods, you would have plenty of bone-boosting calcium for the day. Learn to read labels, and make sure your calcium intake equals the recommended requirements for keeping bones strong (page 19).

93. Throw in chunks of fresh vegetables and tofu if you are using a prepared pasta sauce. Grated carrots, sliced onions and peppers, and chopped zucchini are excellent bone-boosting foods and make any sauce taste richer.

94. Plantains are filled with vitamins A and C. They are best when the outer peel is turning black. Peel and slice the plantain, then sauté in 1 tablespoon butter and serve with honey or powdered sugar.

95. Toss several tangerines into a child's lunch box. This quick-and-easy snack provides half of your daily vitamin C requirement

96. Two tablespoons of dried fruit counts as one serving of fruits and vegetables. Keep a bowl of dried fruit around for a quick-and-easy bone-boosting snack.

97. Fat-free Parmesan cheese is a great bone-boosting alternative to some of the higher fat cheeses used in recipes. While you may have to get used to the taste, you will benefit from the bone-boosting calcium and zero fat.

98. Endive lettuce pulled apart into single pieces serves as a great bone-boosting appetizer. Pipe your favorite spread down the center. Try the salmon dip on page 175 for an extra boost of calcium.

99. On cold winter days, substitute ½ cup soy milk and ½ cup fat-free calcium-fortified milk for each cup of water when making a hot oatmeal or cream of wheat. Serve with fresh fruit and whole grain bread for more bone-boosting nutrients.

100. For a quick-and-easy salad, combine 1 bowl of torn romaine lettuce, 1 can mandarin orange segments, drained, and ¼ cup sliced almonds. Use a dressing of 1 part extra light olive oil to 3 parts calcium-fortified orange juice, then top with natural Parmesan cheese.

101. Bake sweet potato sticks for a power source of vitamins C and A. Preheat oven to 400 degrees. Wash 5 medium sweet potatoes, and slice into quarters lengthwise. In a large bowl, mix sweet potato sticks, 2 tablespoons extra

light olive oil, ½ teaspoon paprika, and a dash of salt. Place sticks on a large baking sheet that has been sprayed with non-stick cooking spray. Bake for 45 minutes. Serve while warm.

Section Four

21-DAY BONE-BOOSTING DIARY

Fill in the amount of foods or beverages eaten each day along with the key bone-boosting nutrients. A sample has been given to assist you. Check with the **Bone-Boosting Requirements (BBR)** listed on page 19 to make sure you are getting ample vitamins and minerals to keep bones strong and prevent osteoporosis.

21-DAY BONE-BOOSTING DIARY

	Food/Beverage	Amount	BBR Nutrients
Day 1	milk	8 ounces	cal, vit D, phos, vit A, mag
	scrambled eggs	2 whole eggs	phos, vit A
	orange	1 small	vit C, vit A
	whole wheat toast	2 pieces	cal, phos, mag

	Food/Beverage
Day 1	

Amount	BBR Nutrients

	Food/Beverage
Day 2	

Amount	BBR Nutrients

	Food/Beverage
Day 3	

Amount	BBR Nutrients

	Food/Beverage
Day 4	

Amount	BBR Nutrients

	Food/Beverage
Day 5	

Amount	BBR Nutrients

	Food/Beverage
Day 6	

Amount	BBR Nutrients

	Food/Beverage
Day 7	

Amount	BBR Nutrients

	Food/Beverage
Day 8	

Amount	BBR Nutrients

	Food/Beverage
Day 9	

Amount	BBR Nutrients

Day 10	Food/Beverage

Amount	BBR Nutrients

	Food/Beverage
Day 11	

Amount	BBR Nutrients

	Food/Beverage
Day 12	

Amount	BBR Nutrients

	Food/Beverage
Day 13	

Amount	BBR Nutrients

	Food/Beverage
Day 14	

Amount	BBR Nutrients

	Food/Beverage
Day 15	

Amount	BBR Nutrients

Day 16	Food/Beverage

Amount	BBR Nutrients

	Food/Beverage
Day 17	

Amount	BBR Nutrients

	Food/Beverage
Day 18	

Amount	BBR Nutrients

	Food/Beverage
Day 19	

Amount	BBR Nutrients

	Food/Beverage
Day 20	

Amount	BBR Nutrients

	Food/Beverage
Day 21	

Amount	BBR Nutrients

Metric Conversion Charts

TEMPERATURE CONVERSION

Formulas for conversion
Fahrenheit to Celsius: subtract 32, multiply by 5, then divide by 9
  for example:
$$212°F - 32 = 180$$
$$180 \times 5 = 900$$
$$900 \div 9 = 100°C$$
Celsius to Fahrenheit: multiply by 9, the divide by 5, then add 32
  for example:
$$100°C \times 9 = 900$$
$$900 \div 5 = 180$$
$$180 + 32 = 212°F$$

Temperatures (Fahrenheit to Celsius)

−10°F =	−23°C	coldest part of freezer
0°F =	−17°C	freezer
32°F =	0°C	water freezes
68°F =	20°C	room temperature
85°F =	29°C	
100°F =	38°C	
115°F =	46°C	water simmers
135°F =	57°C	water scalds
140°F =	60°C	
150°F =	66°C	
160°F =	71°C	
170°F =	77°C	

180°F =	82°C	water simmers
190°F =	88°C	
200°F =	95°C	
205°F =	96°C	water simmers
212°F =	100°C	water boils, at sea level
225°F =	110°C	
250°F =	120°C	very low (or slow) oven
275°F =	135°C	very low (or slow) oven
300°F =	150°C	low (or slow) oven
325°F =	165°C	low (or moderately slow) oven
350°F =	180°C	moderate oven
375°F =	190°C	moderate (or moderately hot) oven
400°F =	205°C	hot oven
425°F =	220°C	hot oven
450°F =	230°C	very hot oven
475°F =	245°C	very hot oven
500°F =	260°C	extremely hot oven/broiling
525°F =	275°C	extremely hot oven/broiling

LIQUID MEASURES CONVERSION

For foods such as yogurt, applesauce, or cottage cheese that are not quite liquid, but not quite solid, use fluid measures for conversion.

Both systems, the U.S. Standard and Metric, use spoon measures. The sizes are slightly different, but the difference is not significant in general cooking. (It may, however, be significant in baking.)

Tbs = tablespoon   teas = teaspoon

Spoons, cups, pints, quarts	**Fluid oz**	**Milliliters (ml), deciliters (dl) and liters (l); rounded off**
1 teaspoon (tsp)	⅙ oz	5 ml
3 tsp (1 Tbs)	½ oz	15 ml
1 Tbs	1 oz	¼ dl (or 1 Tbs)
4 Tbs (¼ c)	2 oz	½ dl (or 4 Tbs)

⅓ c	2⅔ oz	¾ dl
½ c	4 oz	1 dl
¾ c	6 oz	1¾ dl
1 c	8 oz	250 ml (or ¼ L)

Spoons, cups, pints, quarts	Fluid oz	Milliliters (ml), deciliters (dl) and liters (l); rounded off
2 c (1 pint)	16 oz	500 ml (or ½ L)
4 c (1 quart)	32 oz	1 L
4 qt (1 gallon)	128 oz	3¾ L

Solid Measures Conversion

Converting solid measures between U.S. standard and metrics is not as straightforward as it might seem. The density of the substance being measured makes a big difference in the volume to weight conversion. For example, 1 tablespoon of flour is ¼ ounce and 8.75 grams whereas 1 tablespoon of butter or shortening is ½ ounce and 15 grams. The following chart is intended as a guide only, some experimentation may be necessary to achieve success.

Formulas for conversion
  ounces to grams: multiply ounces by 28.35
  grams to ounces: multiply grams figure by .035

ounces	pounds	grams	kilograms
1		30	
4	¼	115	
8	½	225	
9		250	¼
12	¾	430	
16	1	450	
18		500	½
	2¼	1000	1
	5		2¼
	10		4½

LINEAR MEASURES CONVERSION

Pan sizes are very different in countries that use metrics versus the U.S. standard. This is more significant in baking than in general cooking.

Formulas for conversion
   inches to centimeters: multiply the inch by 2.54
   centimeters to inches: multiply the centimeter by 0.39

inches	cm	inches	cm
½	1½	9	23
1	2½	10	25
2	5	12 (1 ft.)	30
3	8	14	35
4	10	15	38½
5	13	16	40
6	15	18	45
7	18	20	50
8	20	24 (2 ft.)	60

Parenting Advice

__Baby: An Owner's Manual__ $14.00US/$17.00CAN
By Bud Zukow, M.D. and Nancy Kaneshiro   1-57566-055-5
Dr. Zukow has been fielding parents' most common (and not-so-common) pediatric questions for more than 30 years. From ground zero through the end of the first year, this wise, witty, indispensible book provides answers and practical tips for your most pressing problems.

__How to Get the Best Public Education for Your Child__
A Practical Parent's Guide for the 1990's $4.50US/$5.50CAN
By Carol A. Ryan & Paula Sline with Barbara Lagowski   0-8217-4038-5
Here is an insider's perspective combining general information with specific advice. The book includes how to select the best school for your child, how to judge your child's progress, and how to evaluate their teachers. Written by two authors with over 40 years of combined experience in education, this guide will help children fulfill their potential.

__Stepparenting__
Everything You Need to Know to Make it Work $13.00US/$16.00CAN
By Jeanette Lofas, CSW, with Dawn B. Sova   1-57566-113-6
Practical, current advice for dealing with the many baffling issues that beset today's stepfamilies. From dating to remarriage, from stepsibling rivalry to joint custody, here is an invaluable resource for coping with today's most complex challenges. Discover the techniques, tools, and strategies that break through the barriers and lead to familial harmony.

Call toll free **1-888-345-BOOK** to order by phone or use this coupon to order by mail.
Name _____
Address _____
City _____ State _____ Zip _____
Please send me the books I have checked above.
I am enclosing $_____
Plus postage and handling* $_____
Sales tax (in New York and Tennessee) $_____
Total amount enclosed $_____
*Add $2.50 for the first book and $.50 for each additional book.
Send check or money order (no cash or CODs) to:
Kensington Publishing Corp., 850 Third Avenue, New York, NY 10022
Prices and Numbers subject to change without notice.
All orders subject to availability.
Check out our website at **www.kensingtonbooks.com**